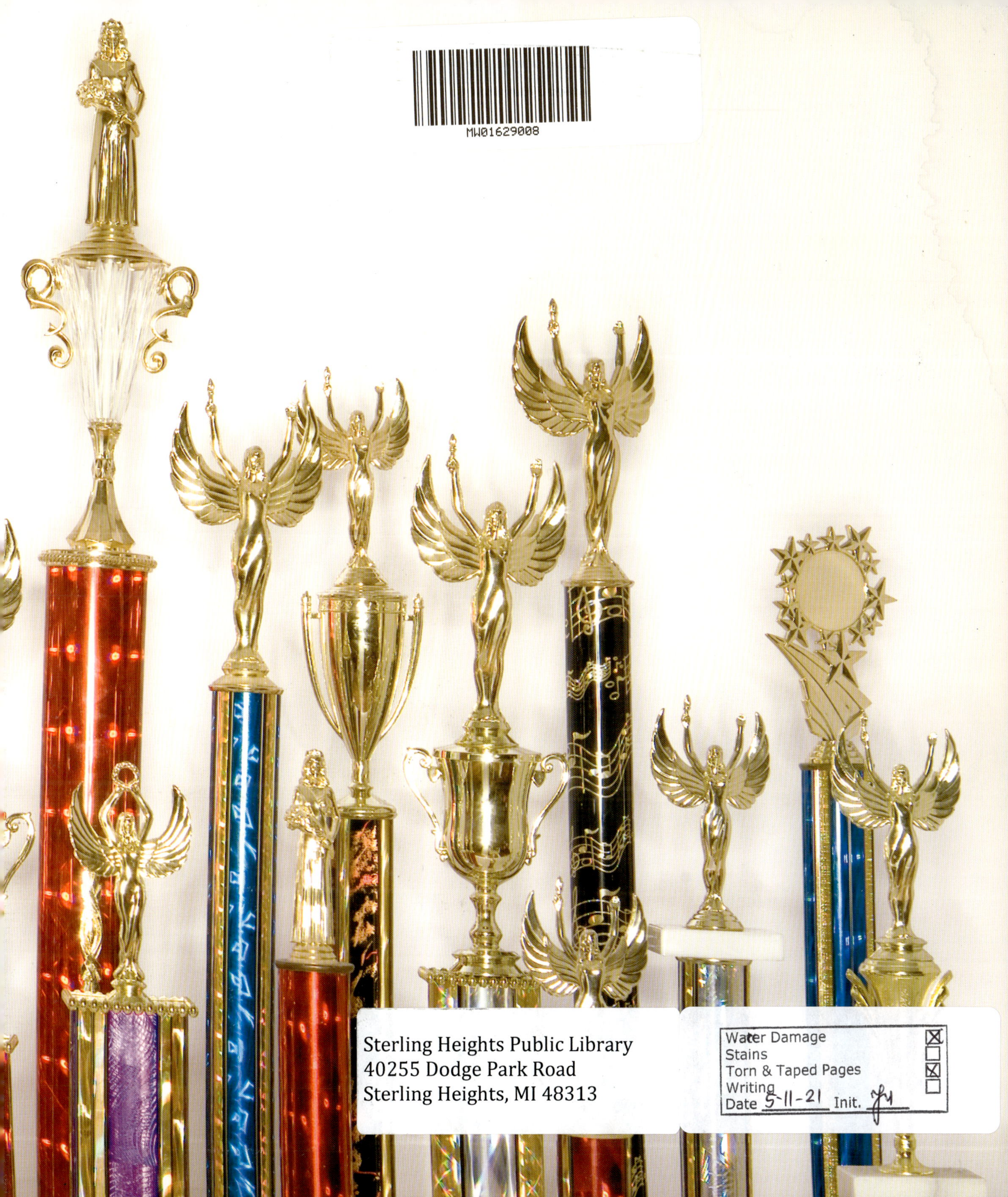

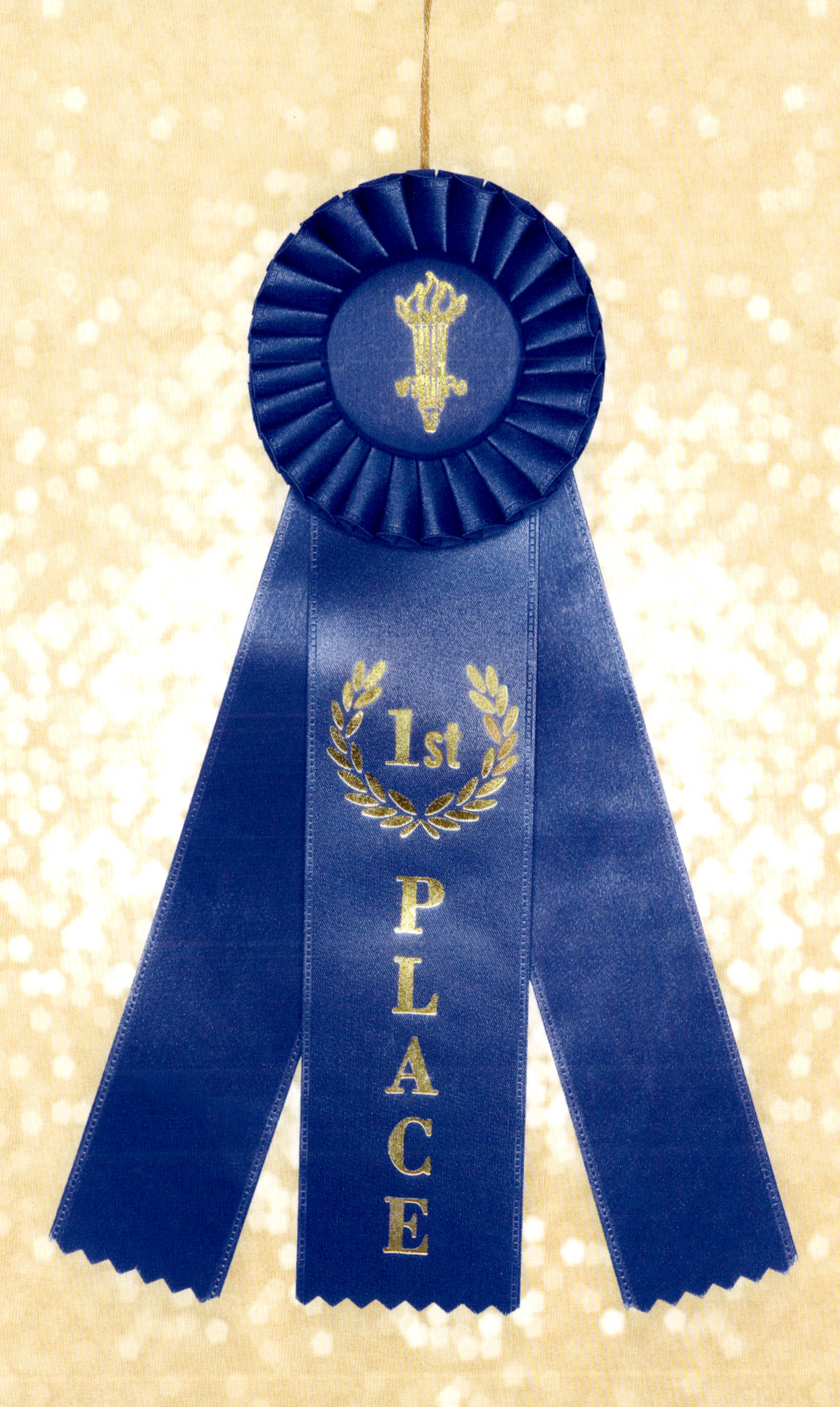
1st
PLACE

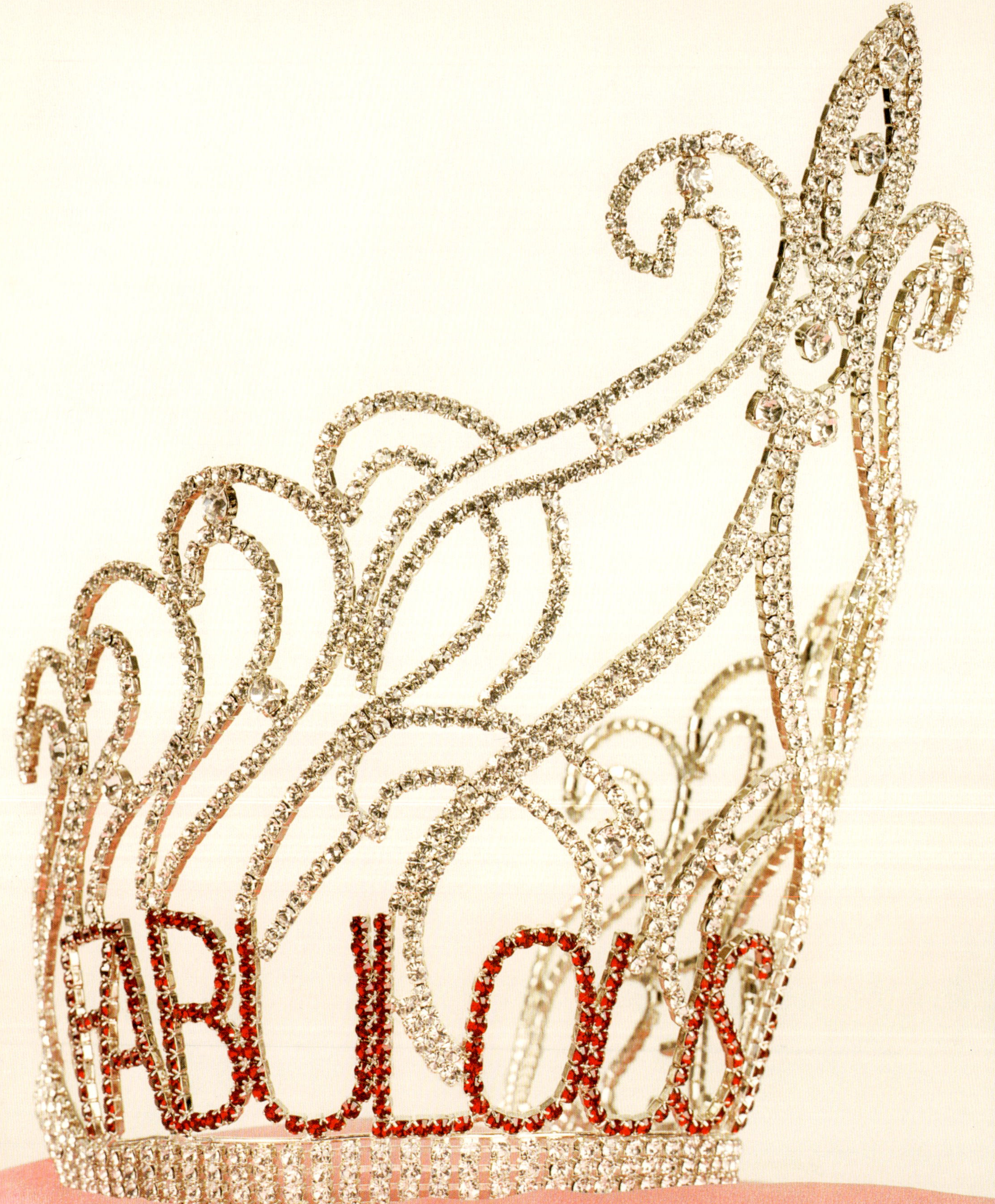
FABULOUS

High Glitz

THE EXTRAVAGANT WORLD OF CHILD BEAUTY PAGEANTS

by Susan Anderson

Foreword by Simon Doonan
Introduction by Robert Greene

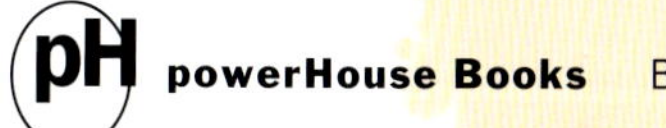
powerHouse Books Brooklyn, NY

High Glitz
The Extravagant World of Child Beauty Pageants

Published in the United States by powerHouse Books,
a division of powerHouse Cultural Entertainment, Inc.
37 Main Street, Brooklyn, NY 11201-1021
telephone 212 604 9074, fax 212 366 5247
e-mail: highglitz@powerHouseBooks.com
website: www.powerHouseBooks.com

First edition, 2009

Library of Congress Control Number: 2009929327

Hardcover ISBN 978-1-57687-514-8

Printed and bound through Asia Pacific Offset
Book design by Liska + Associates

A complete catalog of powerHouse Books and Limited Editions is available upon request; please call, write, or visit our website.

10 9 8 7 6 5 4 3 2 1

Printed and bound in China

Contents

In Defense of Child Beauty Pageants

by Simon Doonan

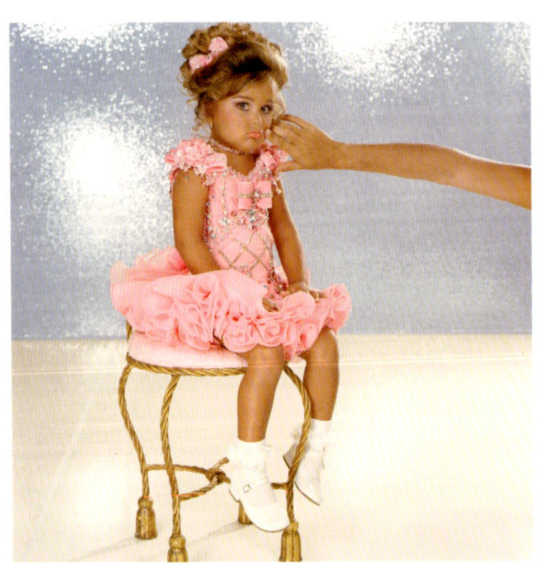

McKenzie ✶ Age 3 ✶ Nashville, Tennessee ✶ 2008

I am totally green! When I look at Susan Anderson's luscious photographic portraits I feel a wave of chartreuse-colored envy. Call me narcissistic, but I cannot help contrasting the show-bizzy lives of these tarted-up tots with my own bleak postwar, scabby-kneed British childhood... and then I become horribly jealous. If only my mother had the presence of mind to teach ME how to bat my lashes and twirl a glittery baton. If only somebody in our house were to have figured out that all I ever wanted was to parade about—like a Madame Alexander doll come to life—in front of a cheering crowd, bathed in adoration and soft pink light.

I realize that my views are unpopular. Nobody today seems to be pro-child pageant. *Exploitive, tacky, sadistic!* The chorus of criticism, jump-started when the tragic story of JonBenét Ramsey brought this phenomenon to the cultural forefront, only gets louder. Child beauty pageants are an easy target. It's easy to watch footage of this strange, sequined ritual and act all disdainful and superior. But seriously folks, are child pageants any more pernicious or manipulative than Little League or cheerleading? The knee-jerk antipathy towards this all-American ritual is starting to bore me. The predictable tongue-lashing meted out to child beauty pageants is clearly coming from dreary, overeducated, middle-class people who have never been intoxicated by the spotlight. And what, pray, is life without a little spotlight intoxication?

Learning to sit still for three hours while your mother's gay best friend re-imagines your hair into a bowling ball-sized bouffant and a torrent of fin-de-siècle ringlets is a skill that is denied the average three-year-old.

Sequins and spotlights aside, there are many glaringly positive aspects to this mesmerizing and haunting ritual. It's time for a rigorous and objective reappraisal:

Child beauty pageants are, first and foremost, a great way to alleviate the brain-mangling tedium of childhood. They are, in both their preparation and execution, magnificently time-consuming. If only the excruciating boredom of my rainy school holidays—running down to the corner shop to buy my mum a packet of fags was the highlight of my day—had been punctuated and enlivened with tap-dancing lessons, tiaras, and tulle!

Child beauty pageants teach endurance. Learning to sit still for three hours while your mother's gay best friend re-imagines your hair into a bowling ball-sized bouffant and a torrent of fin-de-siècle ringlets is a skill that is denied the average three-year-old.

Child beauty pageants teach their munchkin-sized competitors how to lose, and not lose heart. In life, thou shalt not always take home the sequined, Mylar trophy. Thou shalt not always be adorned with the pink-satin sash. Sometimes, sad but true, the pink spotlight points at someone else. Needless to say, I, with my pageant-free childhood, have never learned this lesson. Gimme that spotlight, now!

Child beauty pageants teach social skills. Contestants learn, at an early age, how to share their mascara, and yes, maybe even a squirt or two of hairspray. Deprived of that early pageant camaraderie, I find it hard, nay impossible, to share even the most moderately priced beauty products with others.

Lastly, child beauty pageants are good exercise. OK, so maybe that's a bit of an exaggeration, but, you have to admit, there is no way that sitting at home on the couch watching Dora the Explorer *for the five billionth time burns more calories than mincing up and down a little jerry-built catwalk in the banquet suite of a Comfort Inn in suburban Kentucky.*

Regardless of whether you are pro or con, the proof will undoubtedly be in the pudding: the future trajectory of Susan Anderson's pageant cuties will confirm or deny the validity of their pageant-filled childhoods. Will these girls end up huffing glue on the street corner? Will they become the Amy Winehouses of the 2020s? I seriously doubt it. As with teen beauty queens, the most likely scenario for a former pageant babe entails, at the very least, marrying a local business man, and/or reading the weather on the local news channel, and/or slinging peanuts on a domestic airline. Nothing less, and possibly more: Always remember that Shirley Temple, the primordial glitter from which all child pageant contestants subsequently emerged, lived to become—drumroll—a U.S. Ambassador.

And there, but for my parents lamentable inability to stuff me into a velvet Little Lord Fauntleroy costume, go I.

Artifice and Transformation: The Imaginary Lives of Little Girls

by Robert Greene

We might find the forms disgusting: covering the body with mud, deforming the skull or filing the teeth in Mexico, deforming the feet in China, distending the neck, or making incisions in the face, not to mention tattoos, jewelry, masks, fine raiments, ritual paintings, or even the bracelets made from tin cans worn by present-day Polynesians. The body is made to signify, but with signs that, strictly speaking, have no meaning.

–Jean Baudrillard, *Seduction*

When we see images of young girls in pageants or consider the phenomenon itself, we tend to respond in one of two ways–to moralize or to laugh. If we judge and moralize, it is because we believe that the fantasies revealed in these images are in fact products of consumer culture, reflecting notions of beauty and femininity that are passé and degrading. Perhaps we also envision the mothers behind the scenes pushing their daughters into these events, desperately trying to relive their childhoods. If we laugh, it means that we see all this sparkle and frilliness as irony. These girls are unconsciously reflecting the grotesque side of popular culture and creating camp. In either of these reflexive responses we have the same assumption–the fantasies they create do not come from within them, but are rather imposed from the outside. These girls are merely mirrors reflecting the reactionary, commercial side of our culture.

Let us entertain for the moment, however, a much different possibility–namely that we are the ones who are imposing ourselves on them, that we are in fact responding out of certain preconceptions. Going far back in Western culture, young girls have always been idealized–they are symbols of innocence, purity, and prettiness. Underneath it all is the unstated assumption that they are essentially passive and weak. If we must confront fantasies of theirs–such as those in these photos–that do not fit our ideals of innocence, then we must ascribe it to outside sources. Boys can create their own worlds; their fantasies can be dark and violent, but we can accept the fact they correspond to some desire or need inside of them. Girls are empty vessels, screens of projection; they are not the agents and producers of their world, or so we think. We do not recognize that they could produce something strong, strange, and even freakish all on their own.

To admit that the fantasies revealed in these images come from some place deep within these girls would make it impossible for us to moralize or to laugh. Instead, we would be compelled to understand where they come from and what they represent. This is our task here, but it is not easy. We are not used to treating the inner lives of young girls

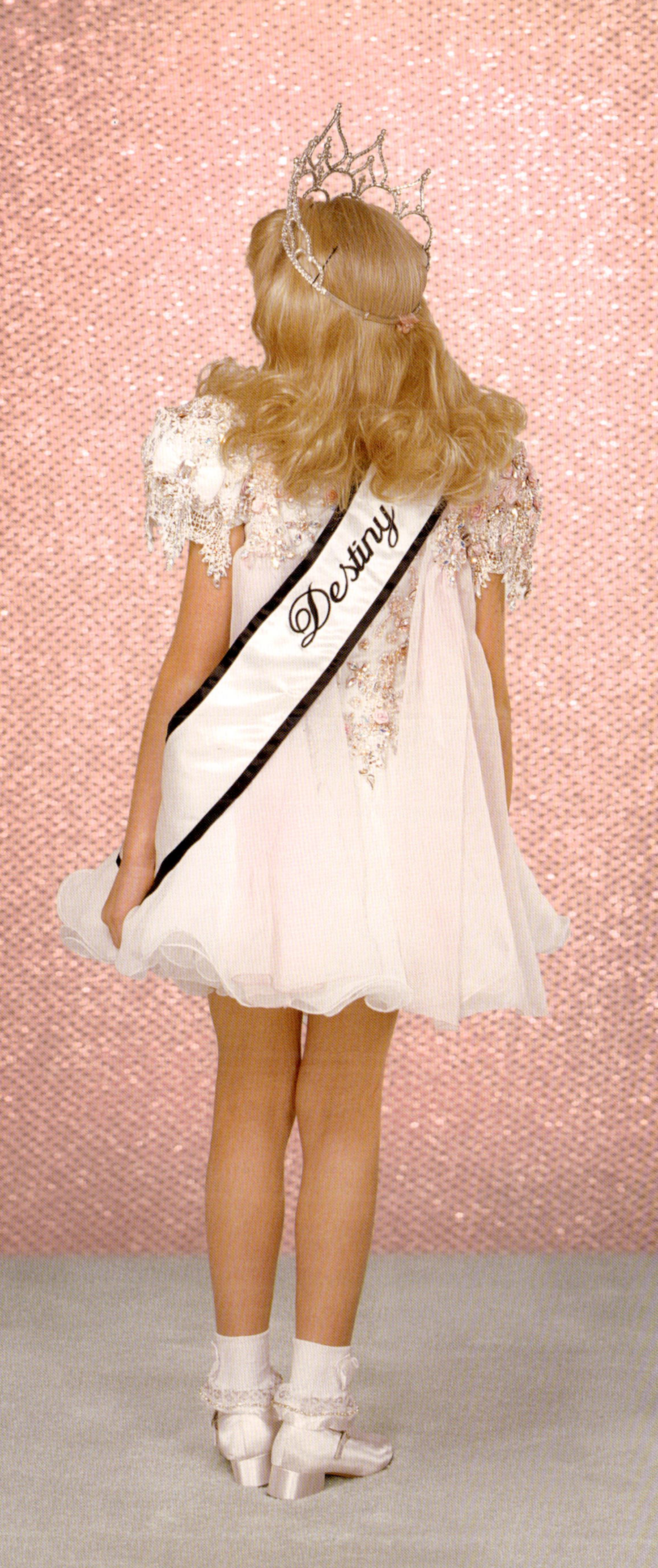
Destiny

But young girls are particularly drawn to the plastic, artificial elements, seeing them as the source of something powerful and fascinating in and of themselves.

with the proper seriousness—as a subject worthy of study and analysis.

In the history of Western literature and thought, only one person has really gone against this grain—Charles Dodgson, known to us under the pen name Lewis Carroll, author of *Alice's Adventures in Wonderland* and *Through the Looking Glass*.

Carroll lived in Victorian England—a world wherein social life was governed by all kinds of rigid conventions and standards of correctness. He was a professor of Mathematics at Oxford University, an environment that was particularly stultifying. Carroll felt out of place among his fellow professors. He was naturally drawn to the world of very young girls, for reasons he could not explain to himself.

In the mid-1850s Carroll took up photography as a way to divert himself from the boredom of professorial life. His favorite subject to photograph was the young daughters of his fellow professors. Portrait photography at the time involved an elaborate process, and subjects had to be prepared to sit for a while. The girls he photographed were singularly uninterested in posing for him and would not sit still for very long. To make them get into the spirit, he had to devise some tricks.

First, he began to accumulate a vast wardrobe of theatrical costumes. He knew that girls like to play dress-up, but he was astonished at the energy and imagination they would bring to enacting various roles before the camera. Second, he brought them into the darkroom, to watch the magical process itself. As one girl later wrote, "What could be more thrilling than to see the negative take shape, as he gently rocked it to and fro in the acid bath?" Third, he told them stories, most of them improvised on the spot. While he set up the camera and the pose, he would keep them entranced with some fable. Carroll was a supremely gifted storyteller, and he was charmed by how the girls would inevitably add to his stories, deviating them in some absurd direction.

One favorite subject of photography was a six-year-old girl named Alice Liddell. Later, on a boat trip and picnic with young Alice and a few others, Carroll would improvise a story that was the basis for *Alice's Adventures in Wonderland* as we know it today.

In essence, Carroll began with a fascination with young girls and the desire to capture their spirit on film. But to do so he had to enter their world, like Alice sliding down the rabbit hole. In getting closer to them in this way, he came to understand the source of his fascination and attraction, and in the process he also discovered two timeless elements in their fantasy lives—*artifice* and *transformation*.

We humans live in a world of complete artificiality. Our language consists of conventional symbols—the word "tree" is of course not the real thing, but an artificial sign that represents the reality. Our behavior in society is governed by all kinds of codes we have created. In our cities we are surrounded by things we have constructed. Our clothes and appearances are not as they are in nature, but determined by conventions of beauty and correctness. We take all of this for natural because it is all we know. Children emerge into this completely artificial world and see it for what it is. But young girls are particularly drawn to the plastic, artificial elements, seeing them as the source of something powerful and fascinating in and of themselves.

In adorning their dolls, they are drawn to colors, clothing, and shapes that heighten this artificial quality. When they play dress-up, they are not doing so to attract male attention for sexual purposes; they are focused on their own bodies and the power they can have to compel attention through artificial devices. They like what is exaggerated, larger than life—colors a bit too bright, shapes a bit too symmetrical, patterns that match in geometric fashions. The girls Carroll studied were all fascinated with language games as well, pointing up the artificial nature of words. They loved puns and anything that detoured our rational world into something absurd. In the tight world of Victorian England, he found them masters at reversing conventions and creating nonsense – a literary genre that Carroll would later explore, inspired by his encounters with these girls.

Transformation is a related power. By donning different clothes, they could enter that particular world of the moment and be altered in the process. Their minds would conform to the image that the costume represented. In this way, mind and body could be transformed. This was the source of deep pleasure and a form of power. It meant the ability to become someone else. The fantasy games of boys often involve such transformations, but for girls it is centered on the body itself, on something physical – in the fetishistic quality of clothes, makeup, and jewelry.

Girls abstract the artificial elements in culture and play with them. They create a world of pure appearances and surface. When they play roles, it is as if to point out the artificiality of all social life – adults are like dolls or puppets, acting according to conventions and wearing masks. Taken to the extreme, these roles can be grotesque; to play with them is a form of power. Looked at in this way, young girls are artists in their own right. They are not passive at all, but extremely willful and active creatures. They possess potent imaginations and create worlds that accord to their interest in the artificial.

As revealed in his notebooks, Leonardo da Vinci once had the idea of forging a new visual language, coming up with a kind of grammar book for images, much as we have for words. He wanted to raise visual art from something people glimpsed at hastily, into a form of high intelligence. He could never interest any patron in this project and it lay dormant, a sign of how the visual in Western culture is considered of a lower order. When we see images, we want to put them into words, ascribe to them linguistic interpretations. Art itself has had to become conceptual, dependent on verbal language. Pure appearances and artificiality are subsequently not accorded any serious attention. This includes the world of fashion, one of the most fascinating and revealing signs of the human spirit over time.

In history, the world of appearances has been the domain of women. They have used clothing and artificial means such as makeup to create something uniquely their own. They were the creators of the art of seduction, using appearance to stimulate certain effects. It was their form of power. Seduction operates in a way that bypasses verbal language and operates on the senses. It has its own laws and logic, but at its core is the attempt to avert any kind of meaning. The man who is the target of such seduction is at a loss to say what this piece of clothing, jewelry, or perfume means. Its lack of meaning is its power. It operates against the grain of our culture in which everything is supposed to signify, to be interpreted and judged. It appeals to our repressed desire to explore the non-verbal and be seduced.

Andy Warhol tried to bring such seductive, feminine power to the art world. His goal, in certain periods of his work, was to create pure surface – the references and possible linguistic interpretations flattened into almost nothing by the brightness or shine he created. You cannot move past the surface. It is a similar effect to the images of these girls, who are obsessive creators of the artificial for its own sake, and whose use of shine and brightness tethers our attention to the surface.

What Susan Anderson has managed to achieve with her work in this book is to reflect this surface world – no easy task, and a sign of her artistry. She does not moralize or laugh by creating distance and irony, the usual approach. She reflects. In the process, these images take artificiality to a new and higher level. A photograph, like everything human, is merely a convention. On a flattened piece of paper, certain colors and lines are recreated that our trained eyes fill in and accept as a copy of reality – a photograph.

In these pageant photos, the surface dominates. The candy colors, the highly constructed hairstyles, the elaborate glitz, and the geometric patterns become almost abstract, a blur. These are photographs, no doubt, but they could be paintings or cartoons as well, a disconcerting effect. It is a remarkable re-creation of these girls' fantasy lives, forcing us to see this world on their level – reveling in the artificial.

It can be said that modern culture is moving in precisely the opposite direction. When it comes to clothing, we want things to be comfortable and understated. We prefer looks and manners that are relaxed and informal. Even the wealthy want to shrink into the background, dressing like anyone else. In cinema, we go for muted colors. Technicolor is too garish; it almost hurts our eyes. To us, this represents progress – we are moving away from the fake.

What we have lost in the process is the notion that everything we do is artificial. Our cop dramas and reality shows are merely new forms of conventions that we agree upon as representing reality. They are in fact as fake and constructed as anything else. Our relaxed looks in clothing are as artificial as the world of Marie Antoinette, only less spectacular and creative. Packaged reality is our new form of the artificial. Perhaps the constructed looks in these photos can be seen as a kind of reverse commentary on our world – on our drabness and inauthentic relationship to the artificial. Perhaps it is us in fact who are being judged here.

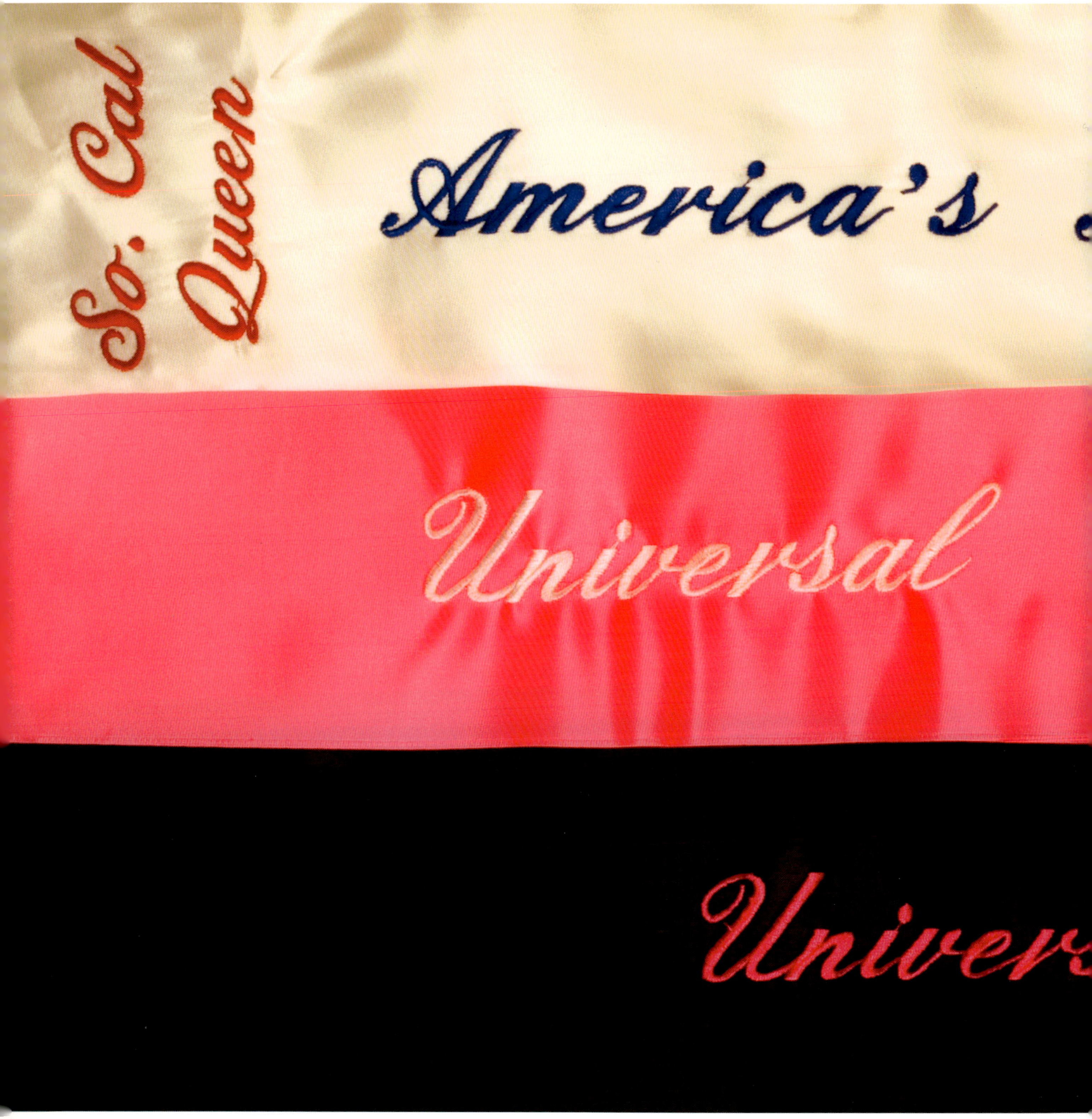

So. Cal
Queen

America's

Universal

Univers

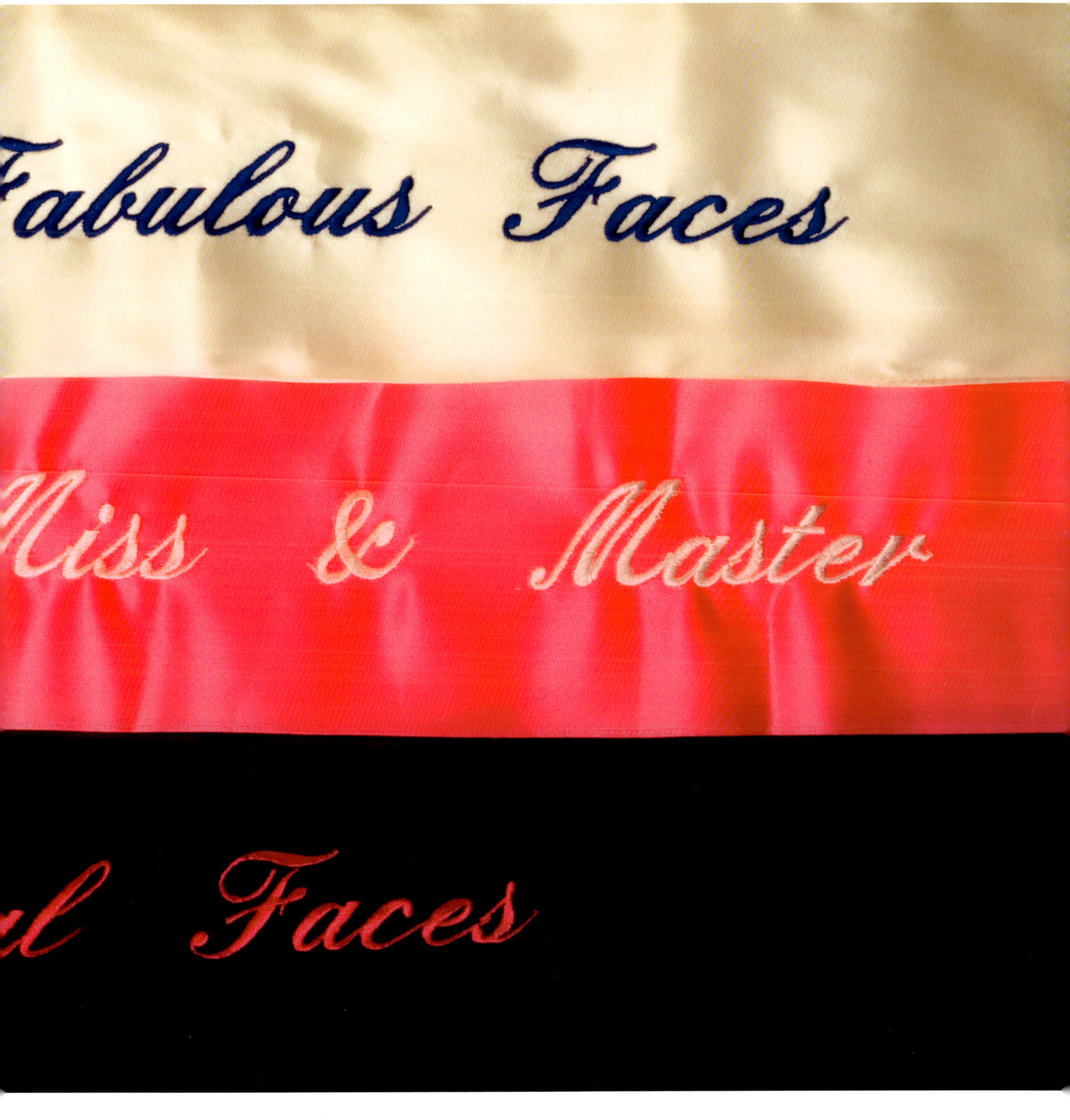

Fabulous Faces

Miss & Master

Faces

Dixieland Dolls

by Susan Anderson

It's Labor Day weekend, and I'm photographing at the 26th Annual Dixieland Dolls and Darlings National Beauty Pageant in Nashville, Tennessee; home of the Grand Ole Opry and musical legend Dolly Parton. For the past three years, I have been photographing children at "High Glitz" beauty pageants around the United States. High Glitz is a particular sub-genre of child beauty pageant characterized by extravagant costumes, hairstyles, and makeup. This pageant, the Dixieland Dolls and Darlings, is rumored to be one of the glitziest, and I can see that it will live up to its reputation.

The lobby of the Gaylord Opryland Hotel has been buzzing all afternoon with arriving contestants, their garment racks overflowing with the customary showy garments and accessories. I take a glimpse into the Tennessee Ballroom and see the Technicolor, fairy tale-themed scenery on the stage. Three-dimensional, gold-glitter-covered letters dominate the set, spelling out *Dixieland Dolls & Darlings*. Legend has it that Justin Timberlake won a car here when he was just starting out. Young boys do compete in these pageants, but my interest for this project lies with the girls who make up the majority of the entrants.

It's Friday night, and the atmosphere is electric as children and their parents line up to sign in for the weekend's events with the sophisticated southern belle Miss Cheryl, school teacher and director of the pageant. My assistants and I assemble my portable studio in the Tennessee Lobby, which feeds into a series of private ballrooms at the hotel, a mammoth Las Vegas-style complex and new home of the Grand Ole Opry. The hotel is part shopping mall/part Disneyland. A Main Street USA-style block is contained within the property, along with multiple theme restaurants, and a 15-story enclosed glass atrium with cascading waterfalls and towering palm trees. Around us in the lobby, vendors set up tables and booths

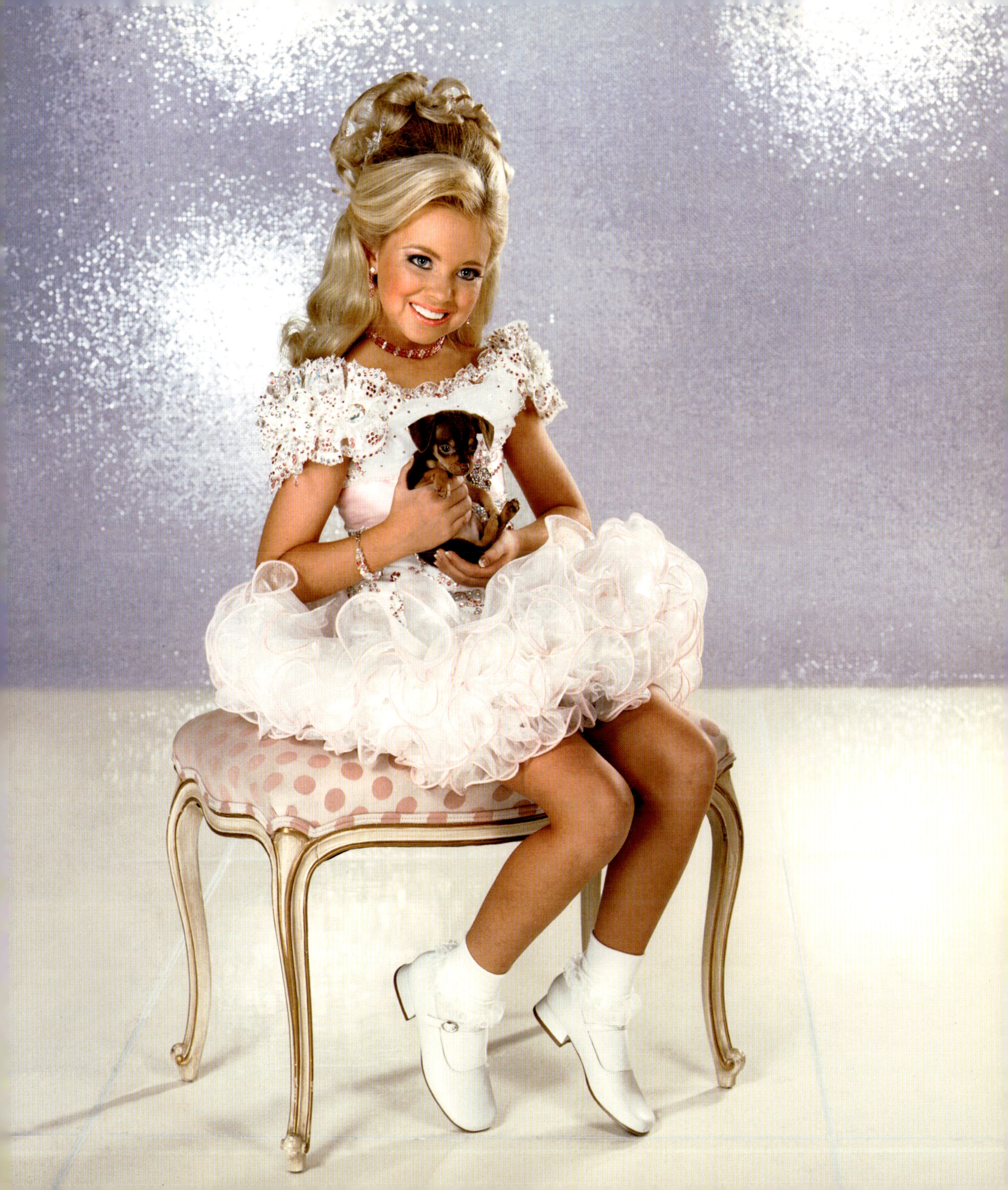

Oftentimes the final pictures look more like illustrations than photographs. The girls have flawless skin, and are spray-tanned, made-up, and groomed to a glossy perfection.

to display the toys, t-shirts, portrait packages, and colorful costumes they will sell to pageant contestants' parents. I purchase two t-shirts, with the words *Total Nockouts* spelled out in rhinestones, as a souvenir. The tops advertise a local group of pageant coaches, who charge by the hour, to give their clients a competitive edge.

We prepare the studio for two days of shooting, roughing in the lighting and testing the equipment. Saturday's events start early, and will include the Sportswear, Swimwear, and Outfit of Choice portions of the competition, followed by limo rides for the participants. Sunday's main event is Beauty/ Formal Wear, my favorite aspect of these pageants, and what I feel epitomizes the visual aesthetic of High Glitz. For this part of the pageant, the girls, primarily between the ages of two and ten, don their most elaborate couture costumes, hair, and makeup. Their custom outfits are encrusted with rhinestones, pearls, ribbons, and bows. From their white-satin Mary Jane shoes and lace-trimmed anklets to their spectacular costumes and towering bejeweled hairstyles, the effect is confectionary.

I have set up some parameters for myself when shooting portraits at these pageants. Rule number one is never to direct the girls other than making minor adjustments to their chosen pose. Frequently I ask to see the back of a dress, or a hairstyle in profile. I make sure they catch the key light just right, or may ask them to adjust a hand, or tilt a chin, but never give any type of creative direction that could be construed as manipulative. My job is to record what I see. The subjects have a self-awareness beyond their years, and have been coached and trained for moments like this one, in front of the camera.

To achieve High Glitz style, countless hours are spent by professional hair and makeup artists on each child. All weekend long, parents shuttle children between rooms off the hotel's hallways, practicing routines, consulting with coaches, changing costumes, and applying the finishing beauty touches. A hairstyle alone can take up to two hours to create. The transformation is remarkable, and oftentimes the final pictures look more like illustrations than photographs. The girls have flawless skin, and are spray-tanned, made-up, and groomed to a glossy perfection. I do very little retouching to the portraits, and it's hardly necessary. Even when printed to the larger-than-life size I create for exhibition purposes, there isn't a wrinkle or blemish in sight – and why should there be?

It's Sunday morning, day two of the shoot, and in an adjacent ballroom Mr. Tim, the Bert Parks of child pageantry, announces the next group of children for the Formal Wear competition to the place he calls *Nash Vegas*. The excitement is palpable as girls mill about the lobby rehearsing their routines, their mothers tweaking ribbons, tying bows, and fluffing ruffles. A father applies dabs of Wite-Out to his daughter's French-manicured fingernails to hide any imperfections, as she waits in the ballroom doorway for her age group to be called on stage.

Pageants are an expensive undertaking. The entry fee, an average of $600-$800 for each child, does not include additional costs such as travel, hotel, custom costumes, professional hair and makeup artists, or coaches. As one parent explained, "They coach them for everything. Coaches will tell you what clothes to wear, which people to buy clothes from, or have clothes made from. They coach all of your talent routines... and you know, while they are your best friend they are also making a buck off of you."

Monday morning, at the Crowning Ceremony, the big winners will be announced. They will receive elaborate 16-inch tiaras and monogrammed satin banners on stage, in front of an audience. Four cars, and thousands of dollars in bonds and titles will also be awarded, followed by Cinderella horse and carriage rides. Talent scouts are known to attend these events, and some lucky child could be signed by a modeling agency. Miss Cheryl makes an announcement that a producer for WE tv is interviewing girls and their parents in the lobby for a new program called *Little Miss Perfect*. The flyer claims *Little Miss Perfect* will tell the real story of these pageant families, without sensationalizing.

Beauty pageants and events like talent conventions tempt little people with big dreams of being discovered by the world of entertainment. Fueled by reality TV shows and programs like *American Idol*, there is an ever-growing perception that there are many opportunities for unknown people to be snapped up out of obscurity into fame and fortune. Talent agent Cal Merlander represents young actors for television and movies. At the IMTA (International Model and Talent Association) convention in Los Angeles he explained his method for finding new clients, "It's just a vibe... It's like the guy who found Lana Turner at Schwab's drugstore. What you really want are the ones who love it up there. You want the ones who live for this. It has to be all about them. And they have to be intelligent. Basically, we want miniature adults. You want kids that look and act like adults and have little adult facial features and little adult mannerisms."[1]

In my studio, ten-year-old Allison sits on a small upholstered bench in the center of the white-tile modular dance floor. She is wearing a white dress with the signature "cupcake" ruffle skirt, and from my angle it almost looks as though she is floating on a fluffy white cloud. Magenta, pink, and white rhinestones embellish the shiny surface, a wide pink-satin sash around her waist. The short cap sleeves of her dress are trimmed in lace, and feature clusters of white-satin roses offset by giant gemstones. Dresses like hers can cost upwards of $2,000, each one a unique couture garment. Her hairstyle, created by a professional who specializes in these sculptural masterpieces, is a combination of her own hair and matching hairpieces. Layer upon layer of blonde tresses cascade down from a vertical crown of curls accented with rhinestone flowers. It's rococo and over-the-top, and from the back it resembles something between a Doric column and a wedding cake.

Allison's mother, Diana, stands behind me, beaming approvingly at her daughter as my assistant makes some minor adjustments to the lighting. She is a natural before the camera, and I patiently watch for the right moment to take the first photograph. After shooting the first few frames of the 12-exposure roll, I hear a tiny voice over my shoulder shouting, "Give her the puppy, give her the puppy." An adorable five-year-old girl, whose sister is a contestant in the pageant, runs up and hands my subject a chocolate brown Chihuahua puppy that will be given away in a raffle at the crowning ceremony on Labor Day.

Allison gracefully cradles the small animal in her flawlessly groomed, French-manicured hands. The Chihuahua is an element I had not considered, but as the tiny dog looks directly at the lens of my camera I realize immediately that it's become part of the picture. The pink belly of the puppy perfectly matches the satin sash of Allison's dress. This new composition is a reinterpretation of an ancient theme: the Madonna and child. Allison smiles broadly, her white teeth gleaming, her eyes tilting heavenward, a vision of optimism and perfect poise. I click the shutter.

1. Jake Halpern, *Fame Junkies: The Hidden Truths Behind America's Favorite Addiction* (Boston: Houghton Mifflin, 2007), 28.

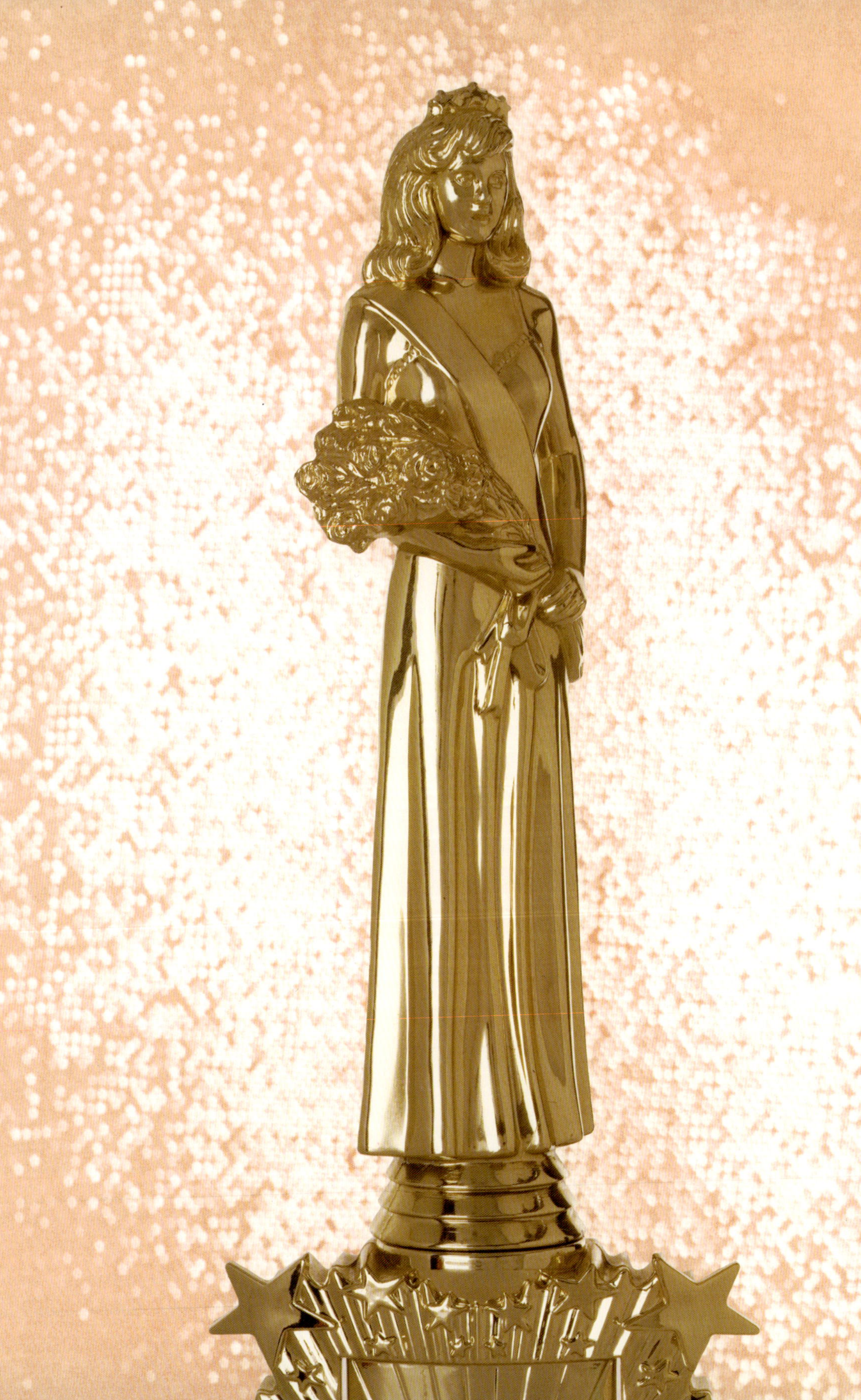

Beauty/Formal Wear

Mary Ashton

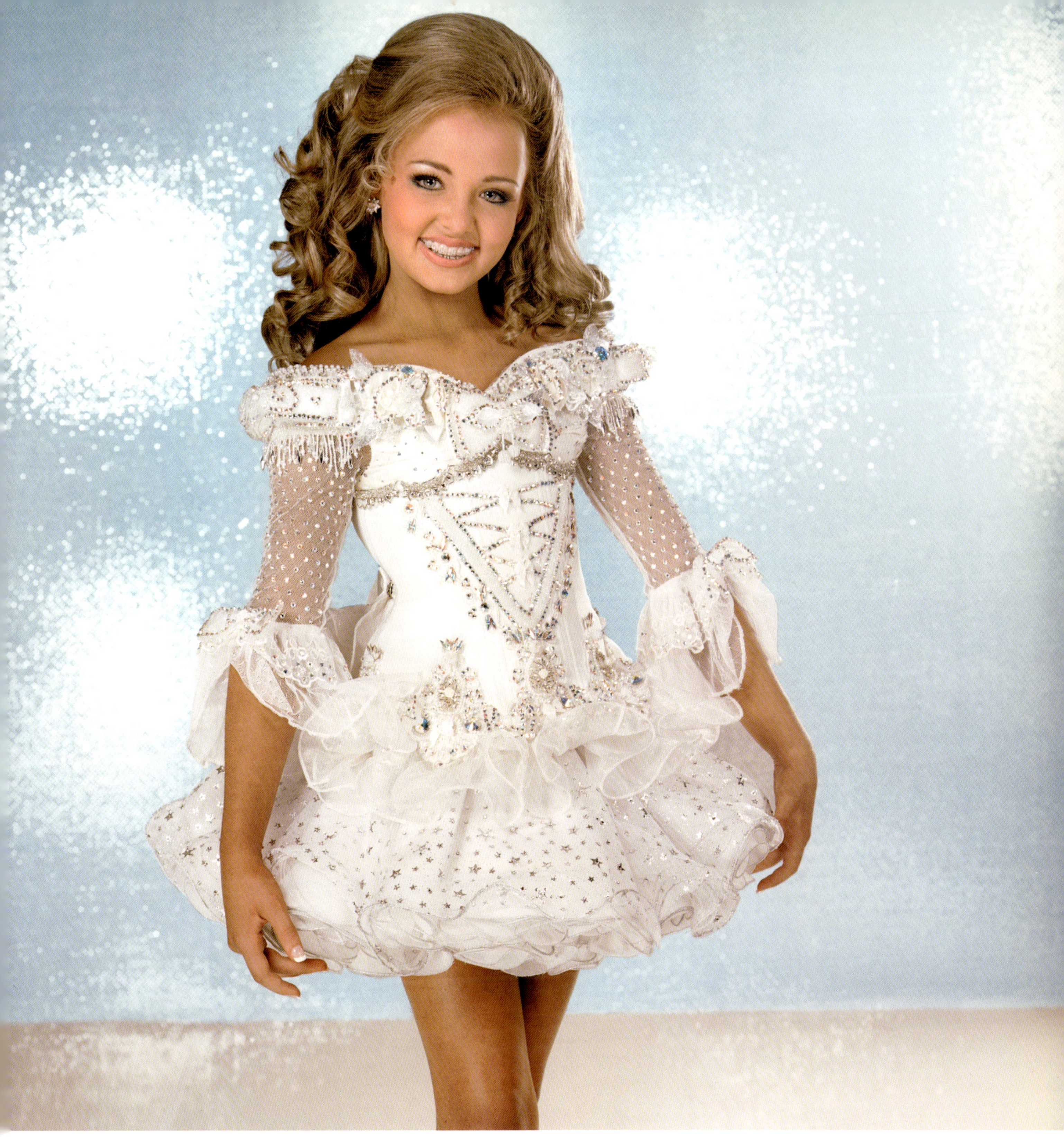

Age 9 ✶ Nashville, Tennessee ✶ 2008

Christy

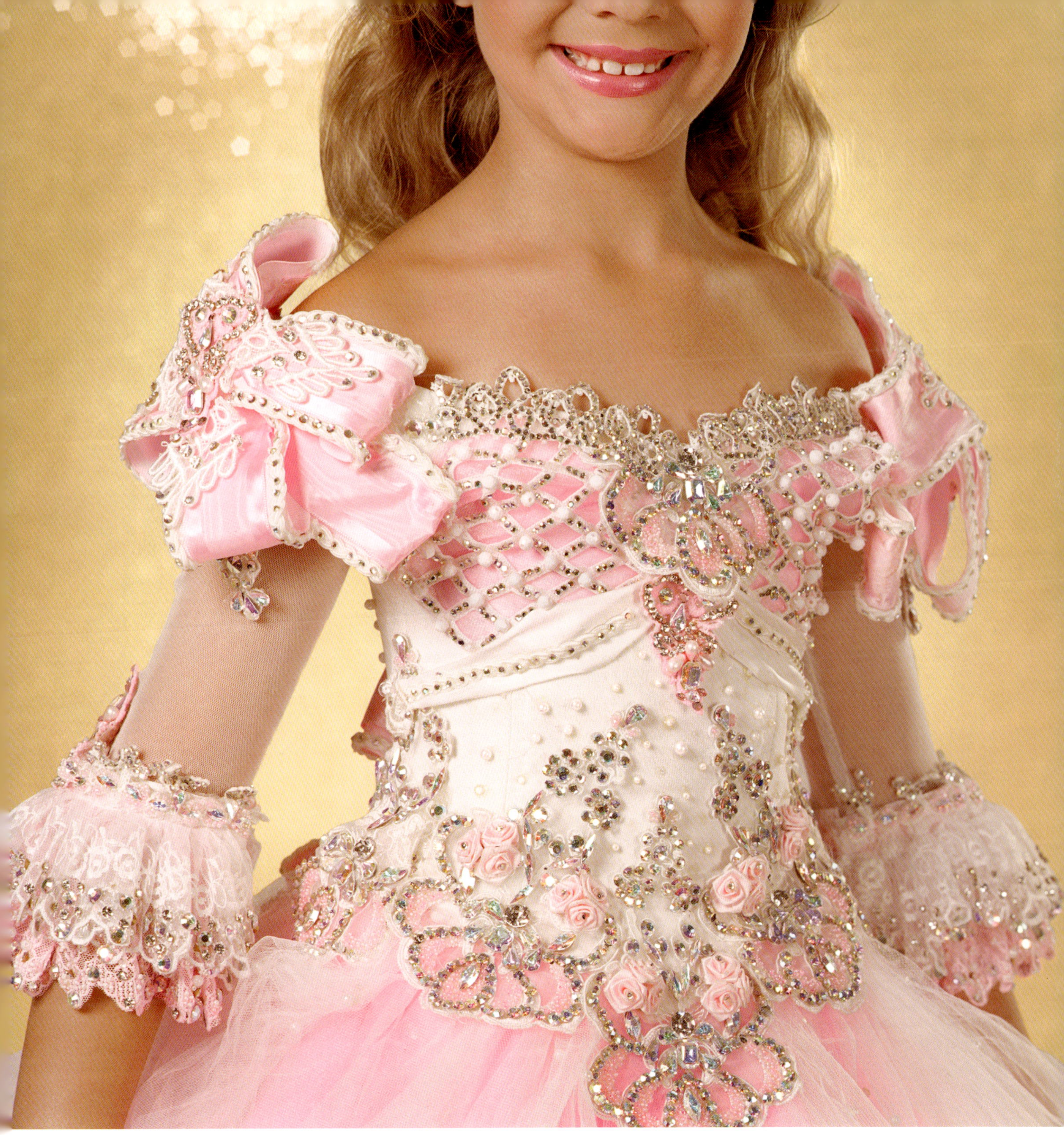

Age 8 × Las Vegas, Nevada × 2006

Kristin

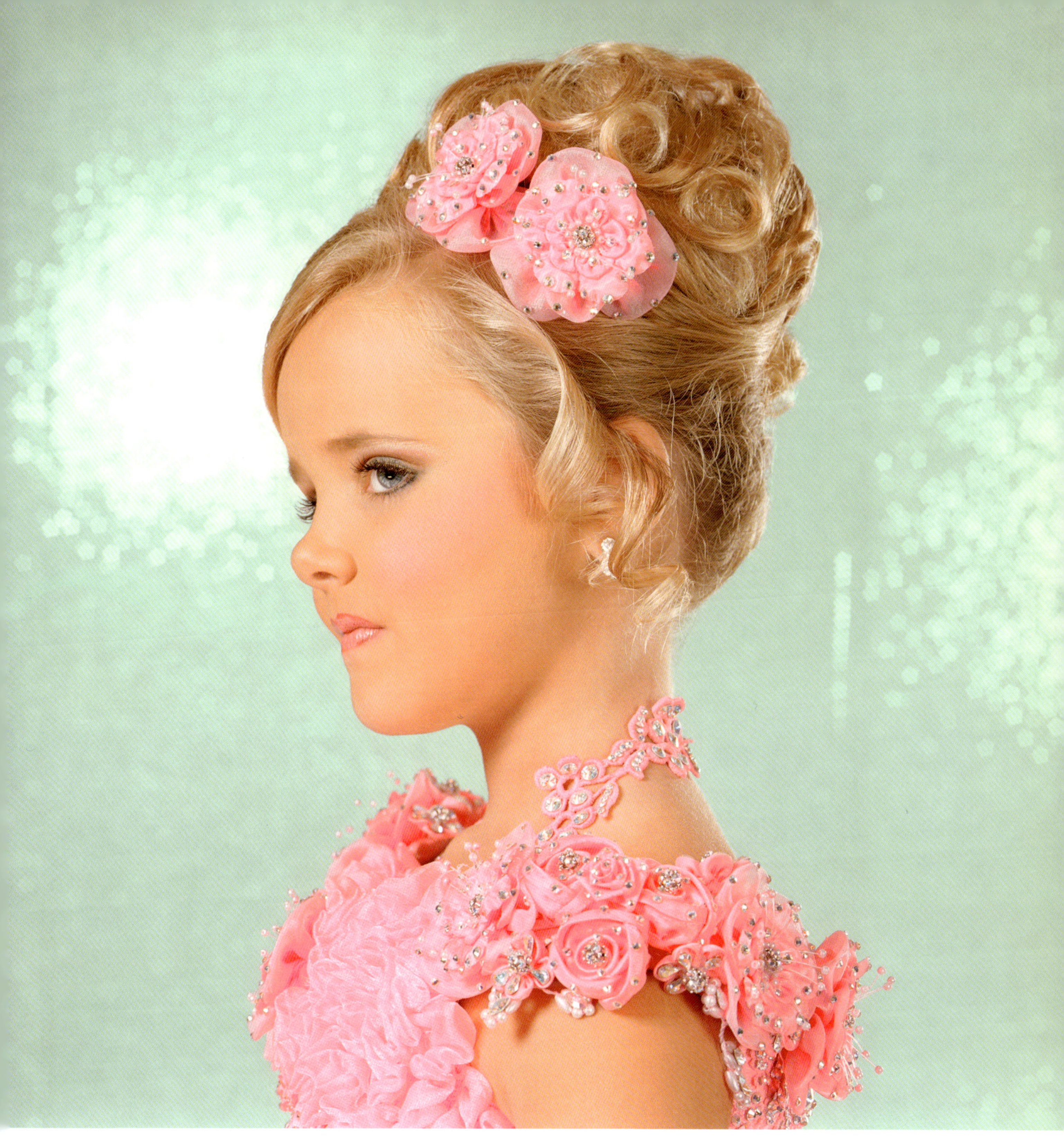

Age 5 × Las Vegas, Nevada × 2006

Tristin

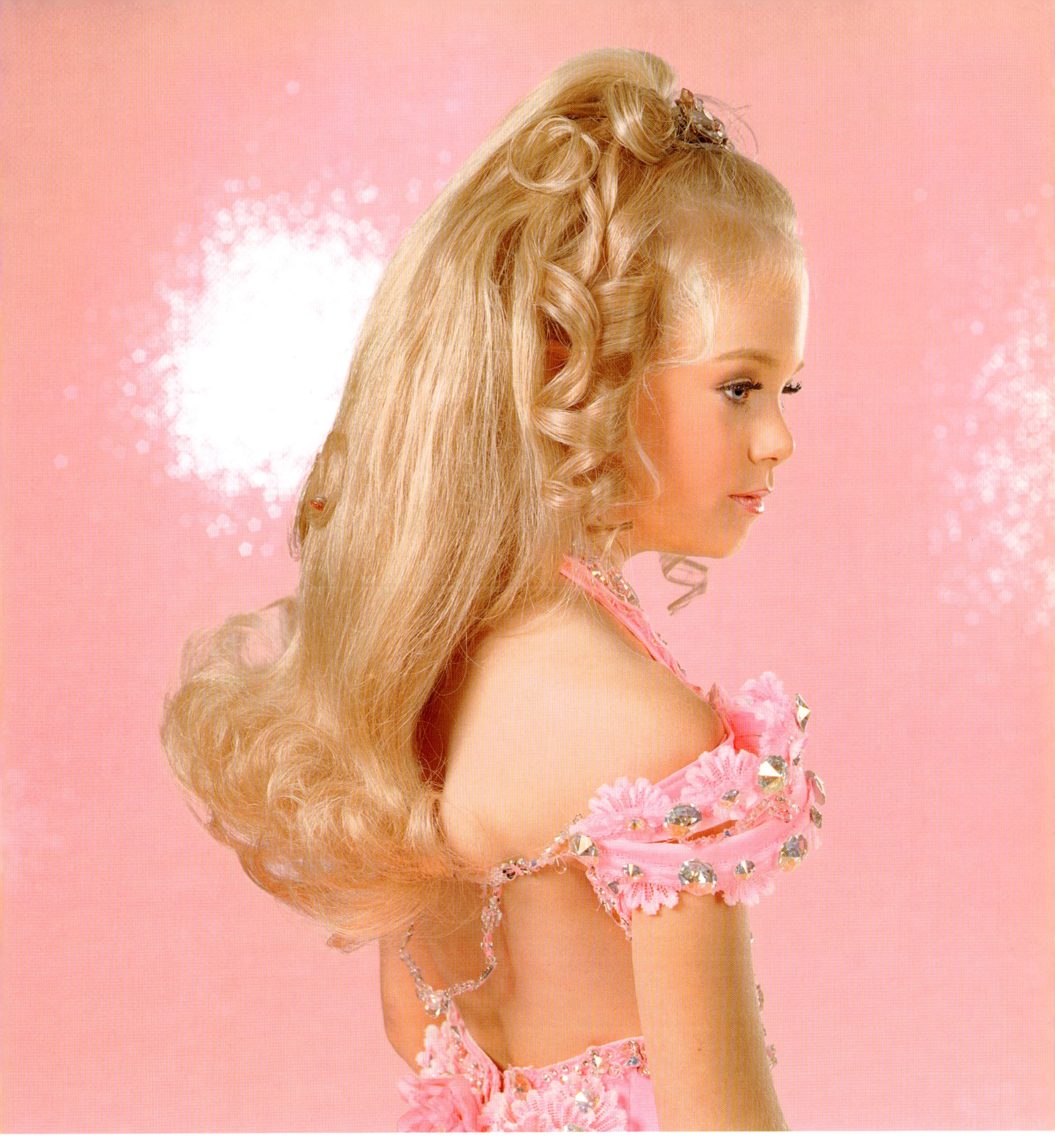

Age 6 × Las Vegas, Nevada × 2006

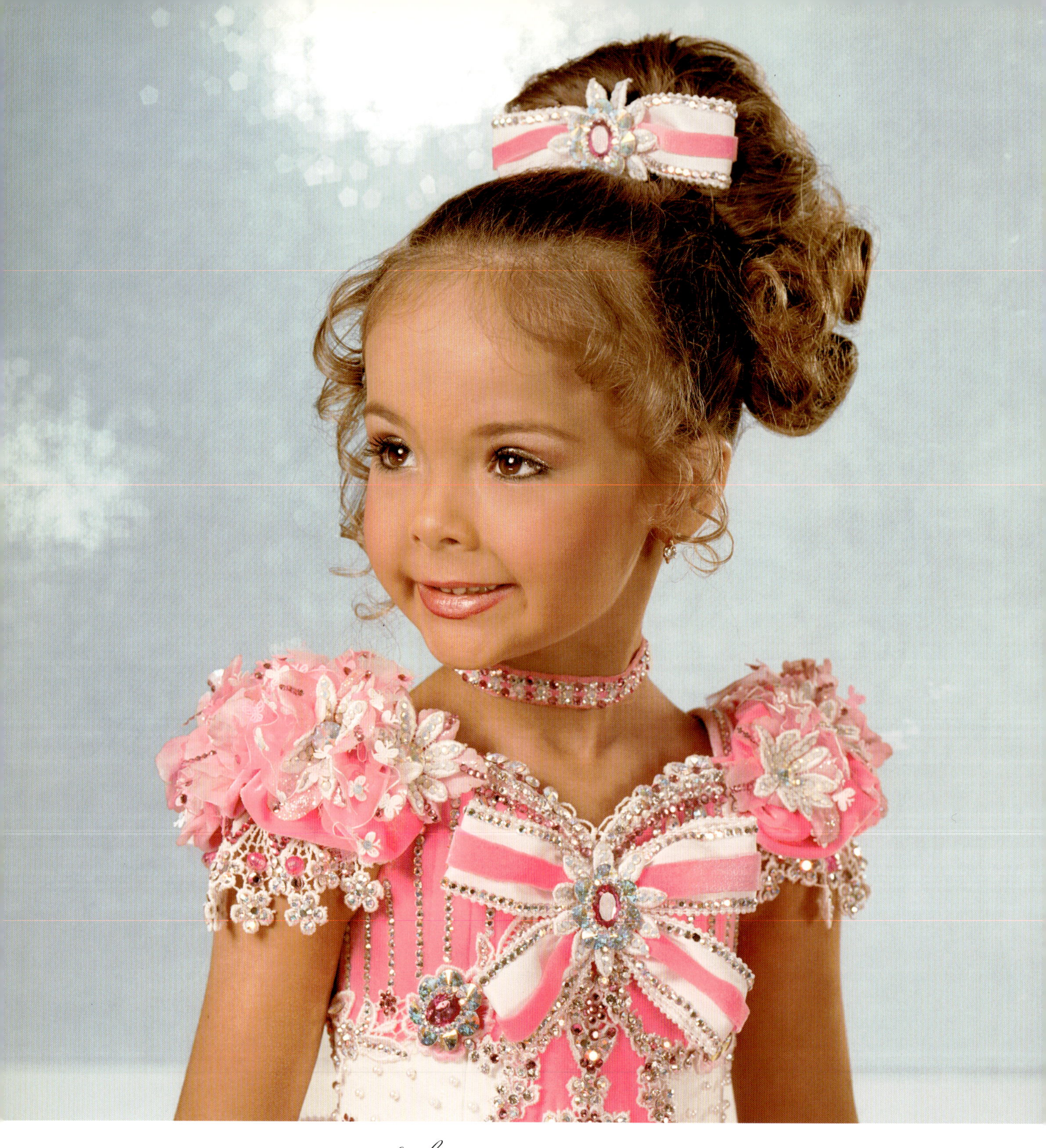

Sasha × Age 5 × Las Vegas, Nevada × 2006

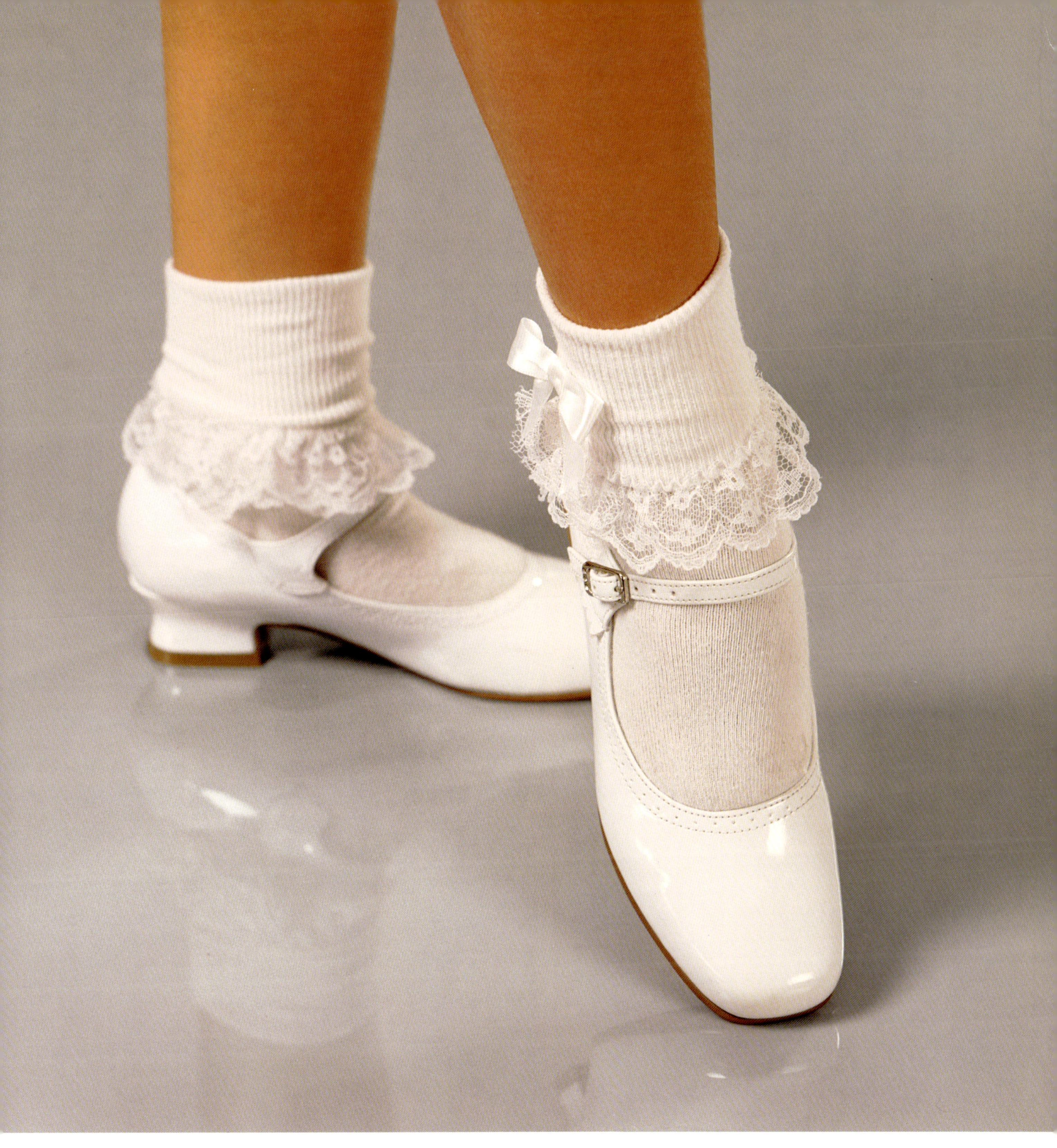

Pretty Feet × Las Vegas, Nevada × 2006

Cameron

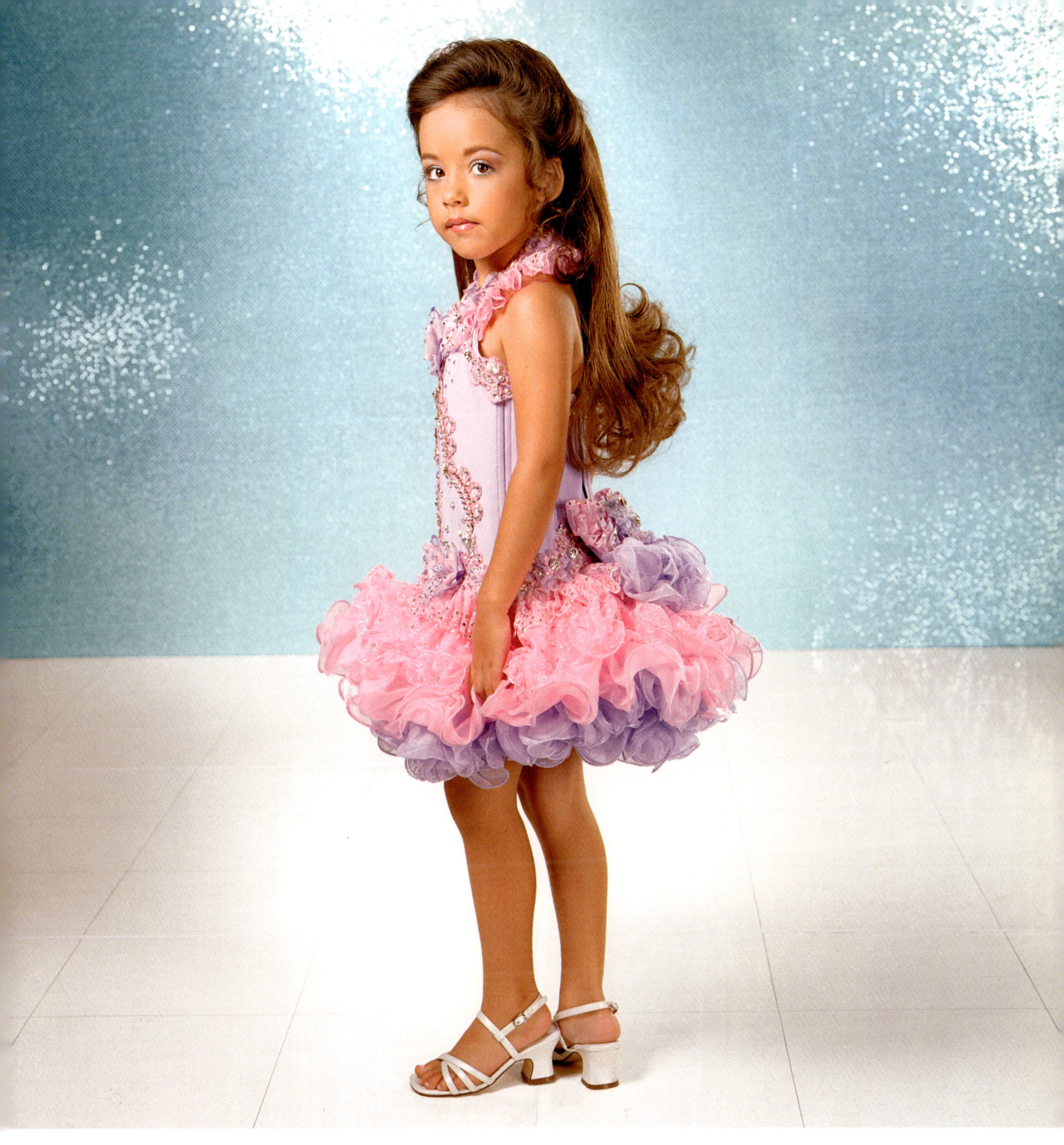

Age 5 × Las Vegas, Nevada × 2006

Elizabeth

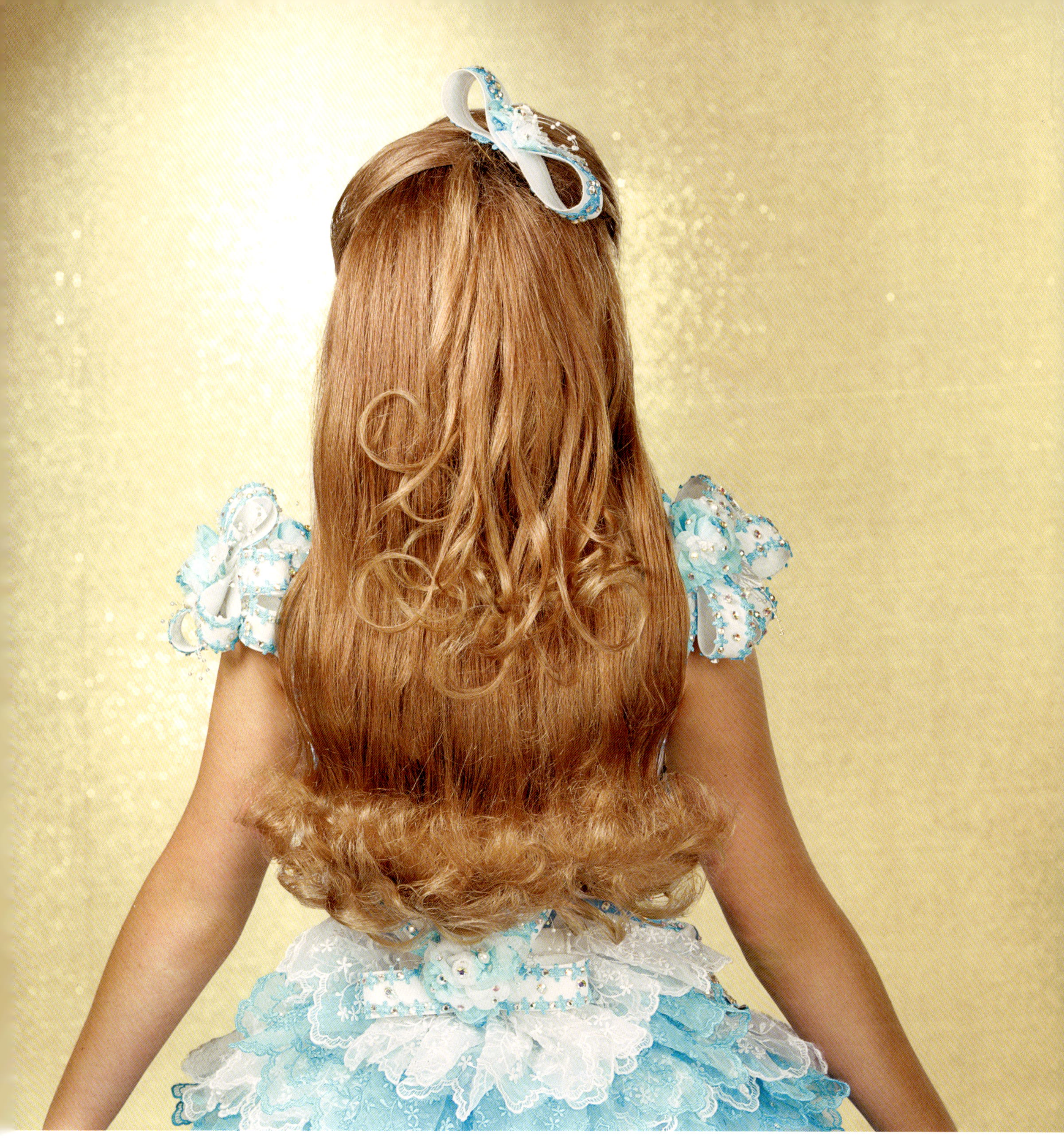

Age 9 × Austin, Texas × 2005

Beauty

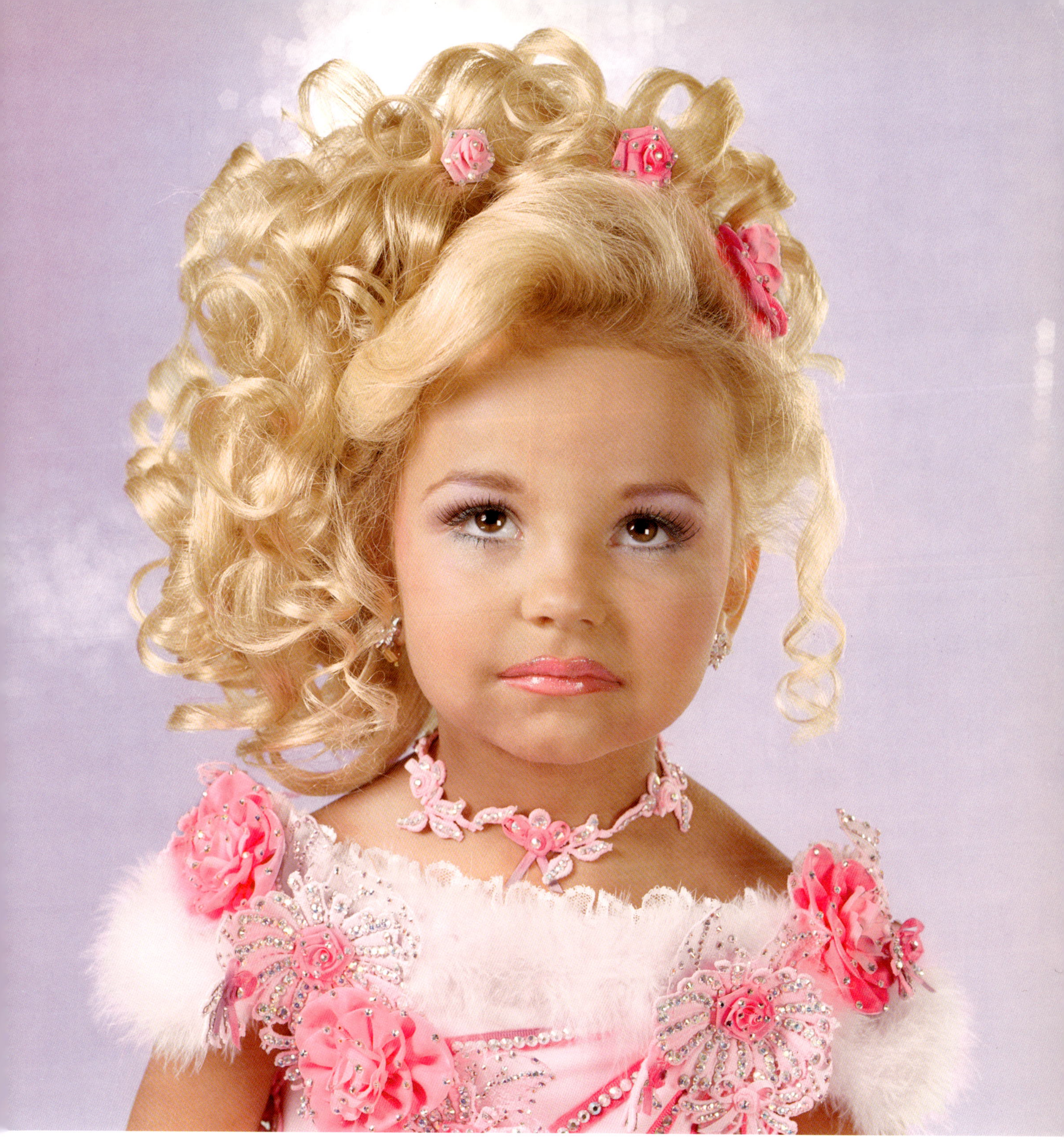

Age 4 × Las Vegas, Nevada × 2006

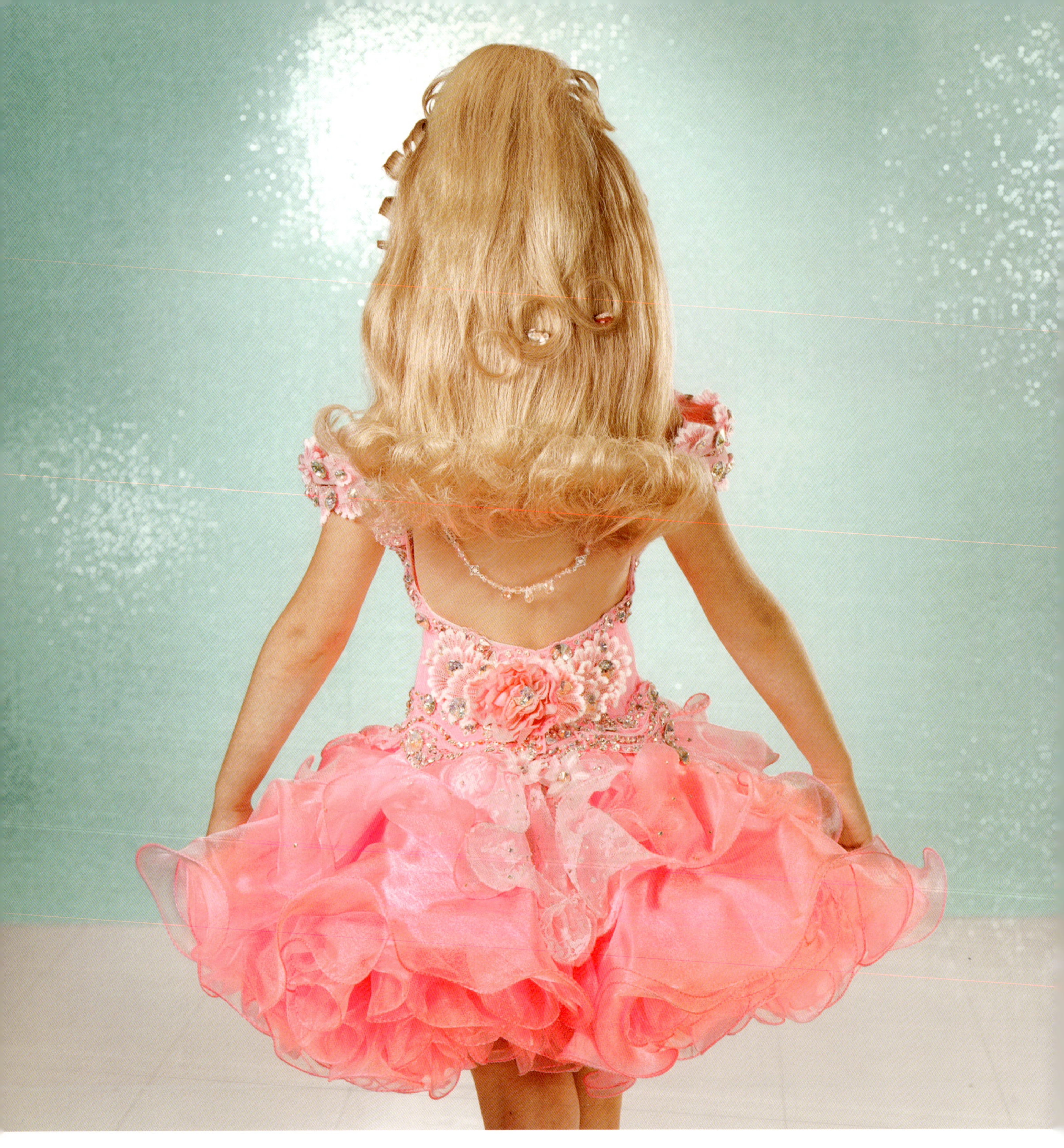

Tristin × Age 6 × Las Vegas, Nevada × 2006

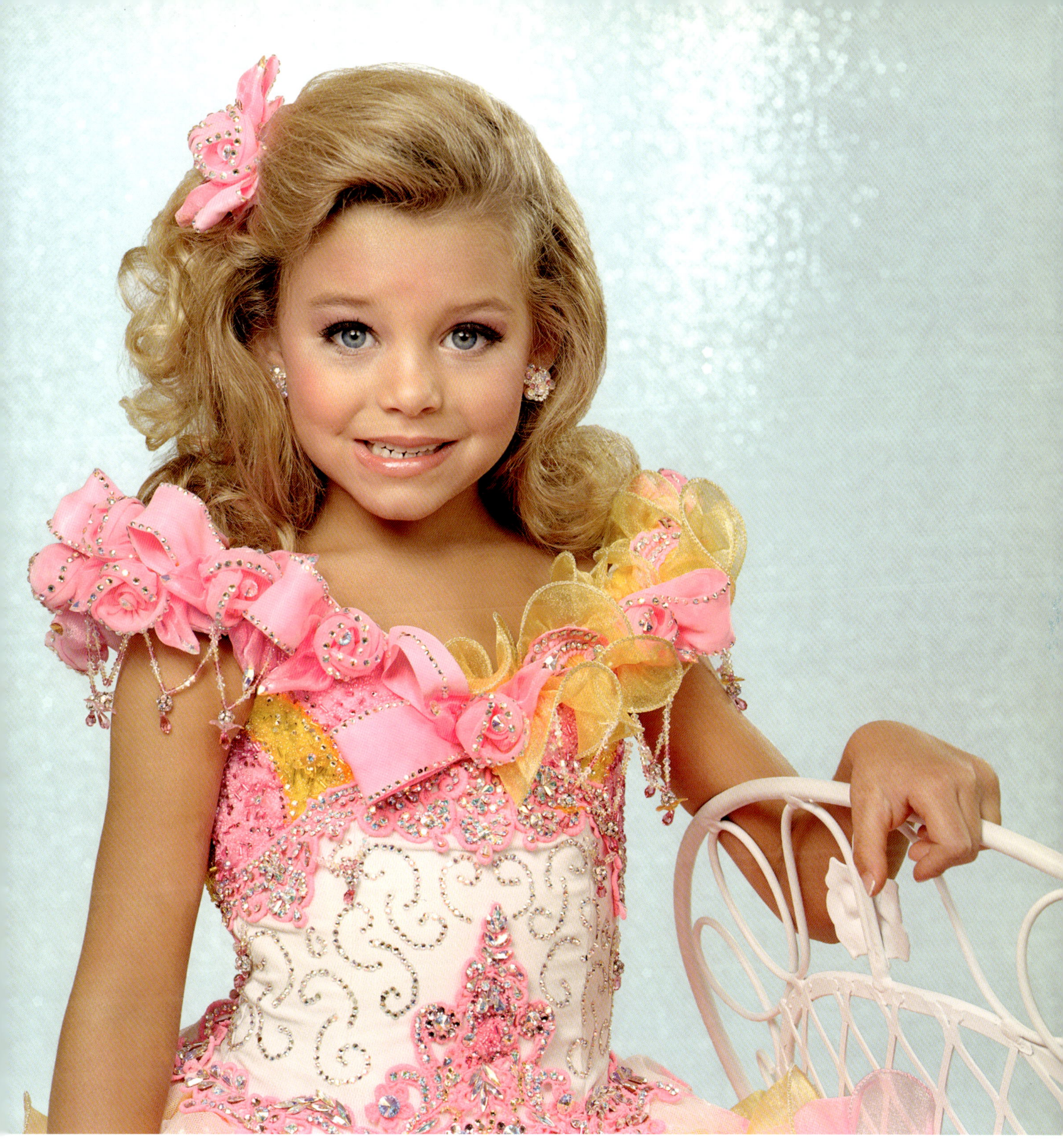

Kyleigh · Age 5 · Austin, Texas · 2005

De Angel

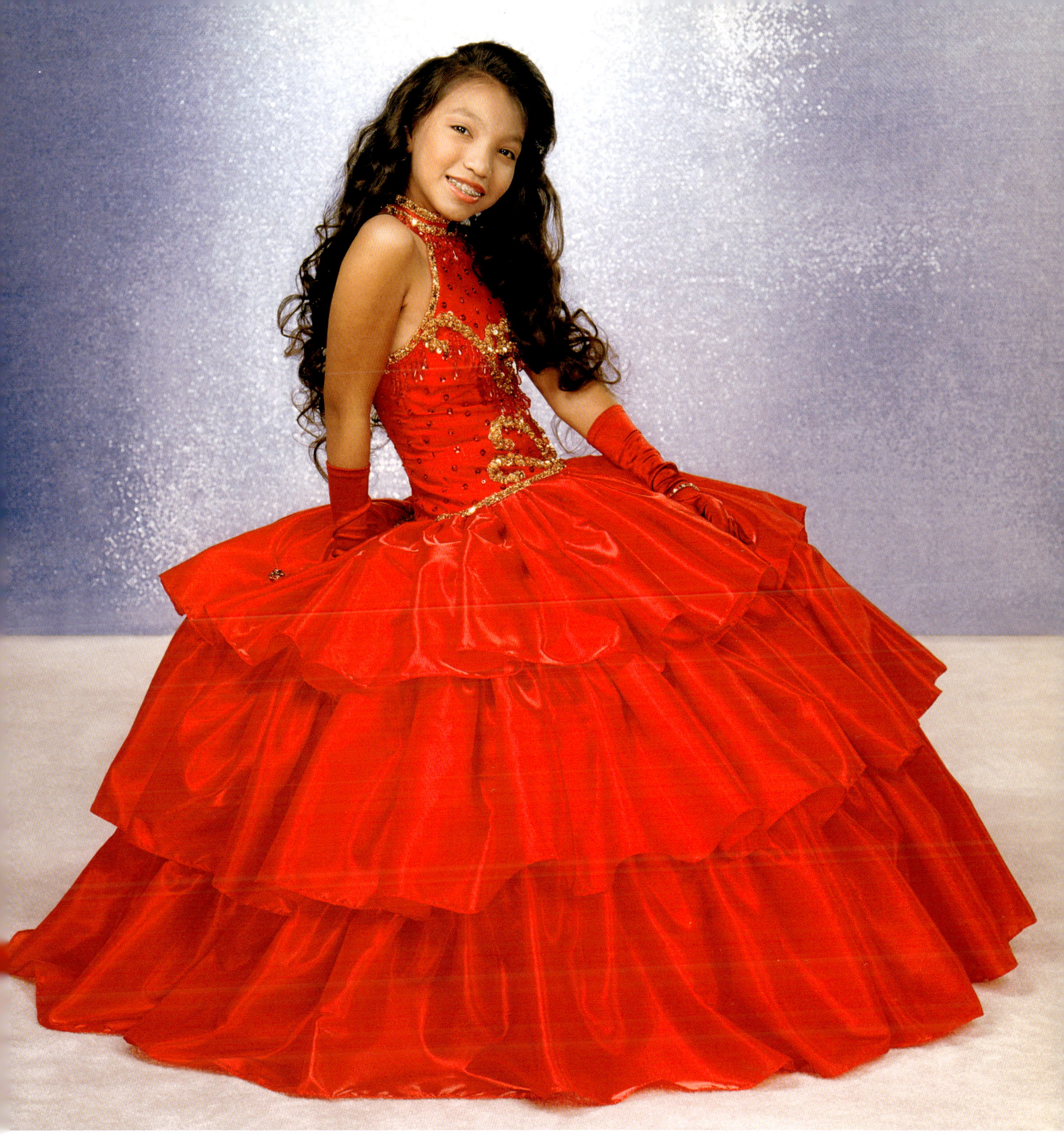

Age 11 × Austin, Texas × 2005

Allison

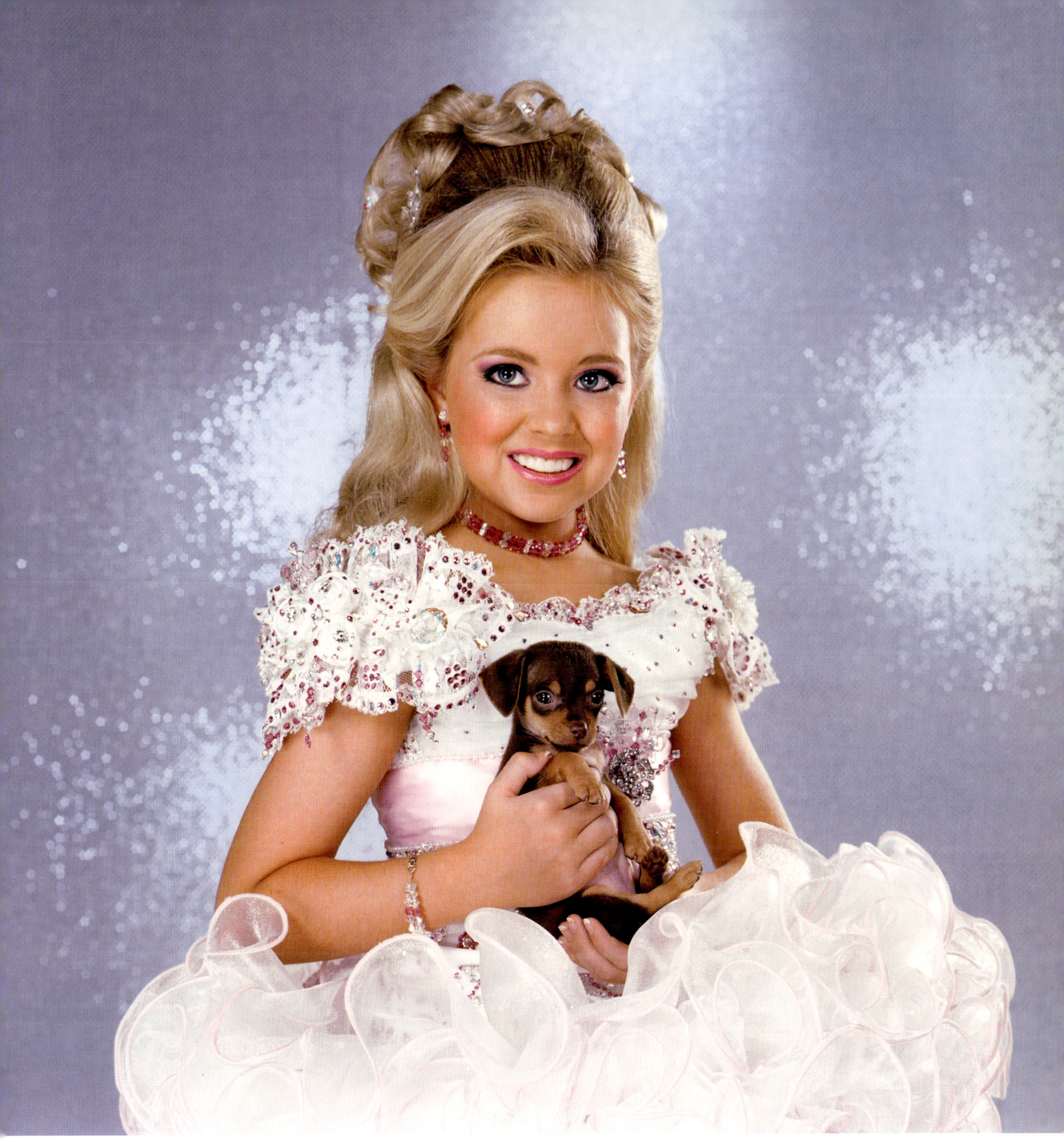

Age 10 × Nashville, Tennessee × 2008

Jordyn

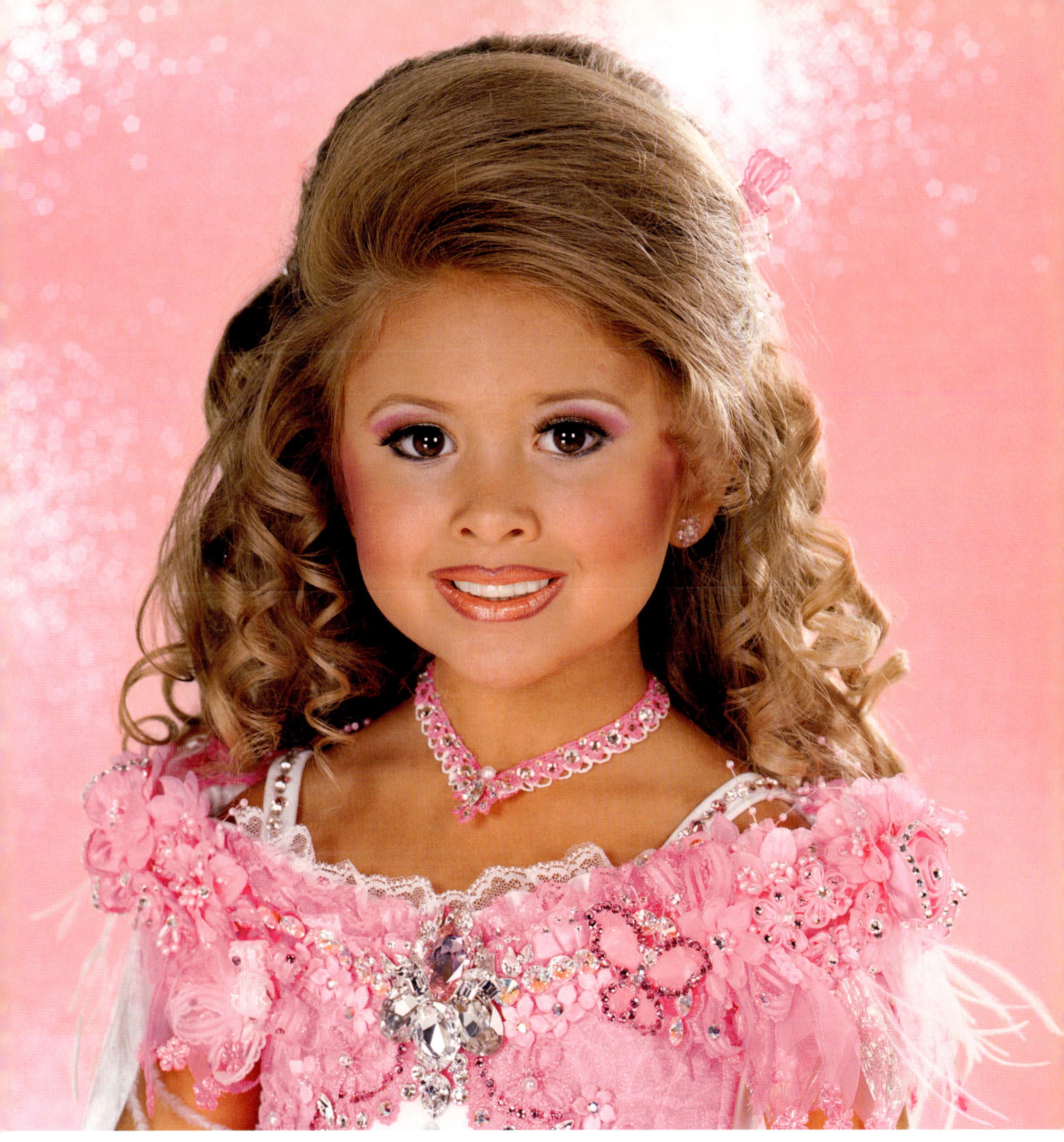

Age 5 × Nashville, Tennessee × 2008

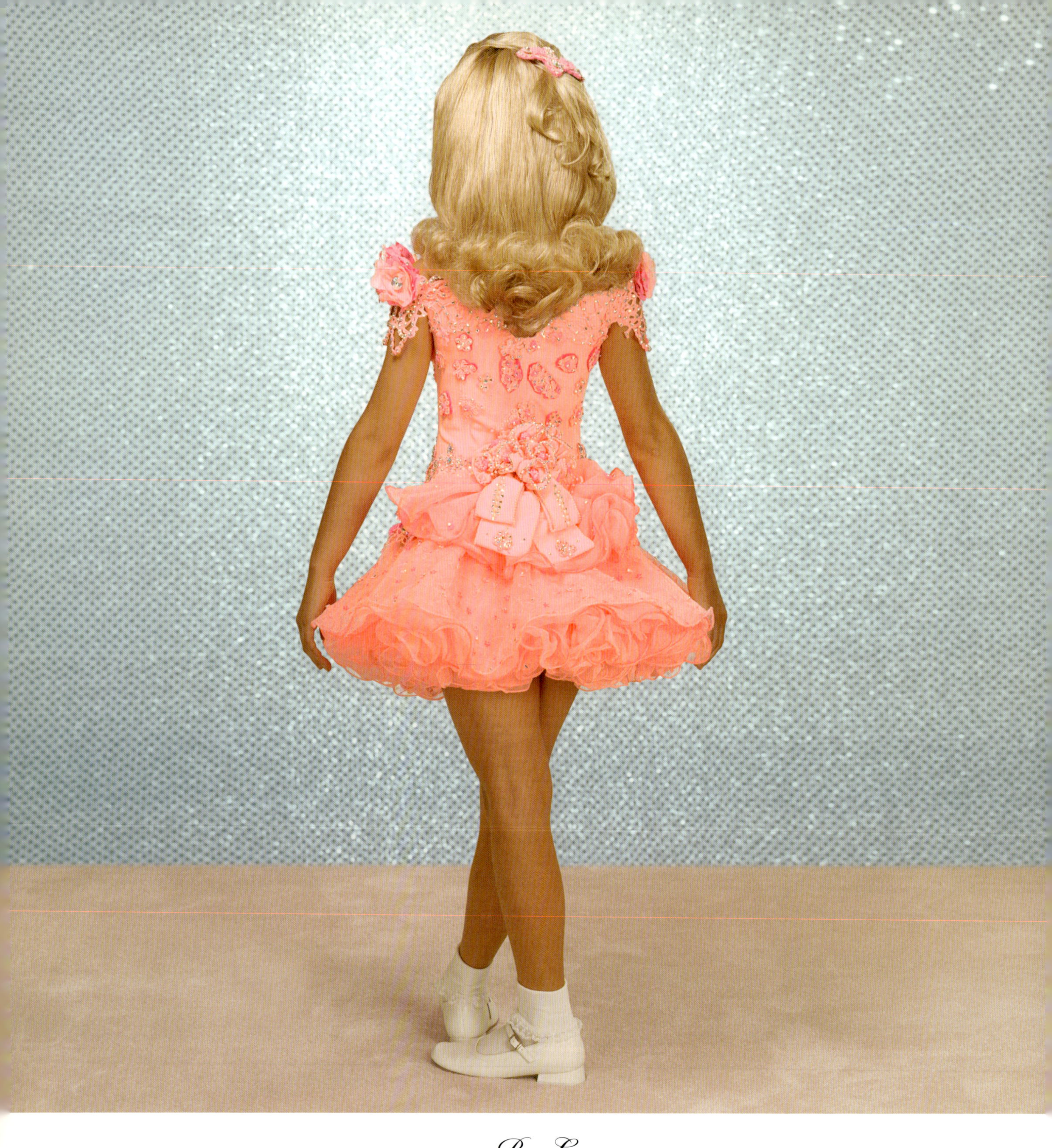

Rae Lee

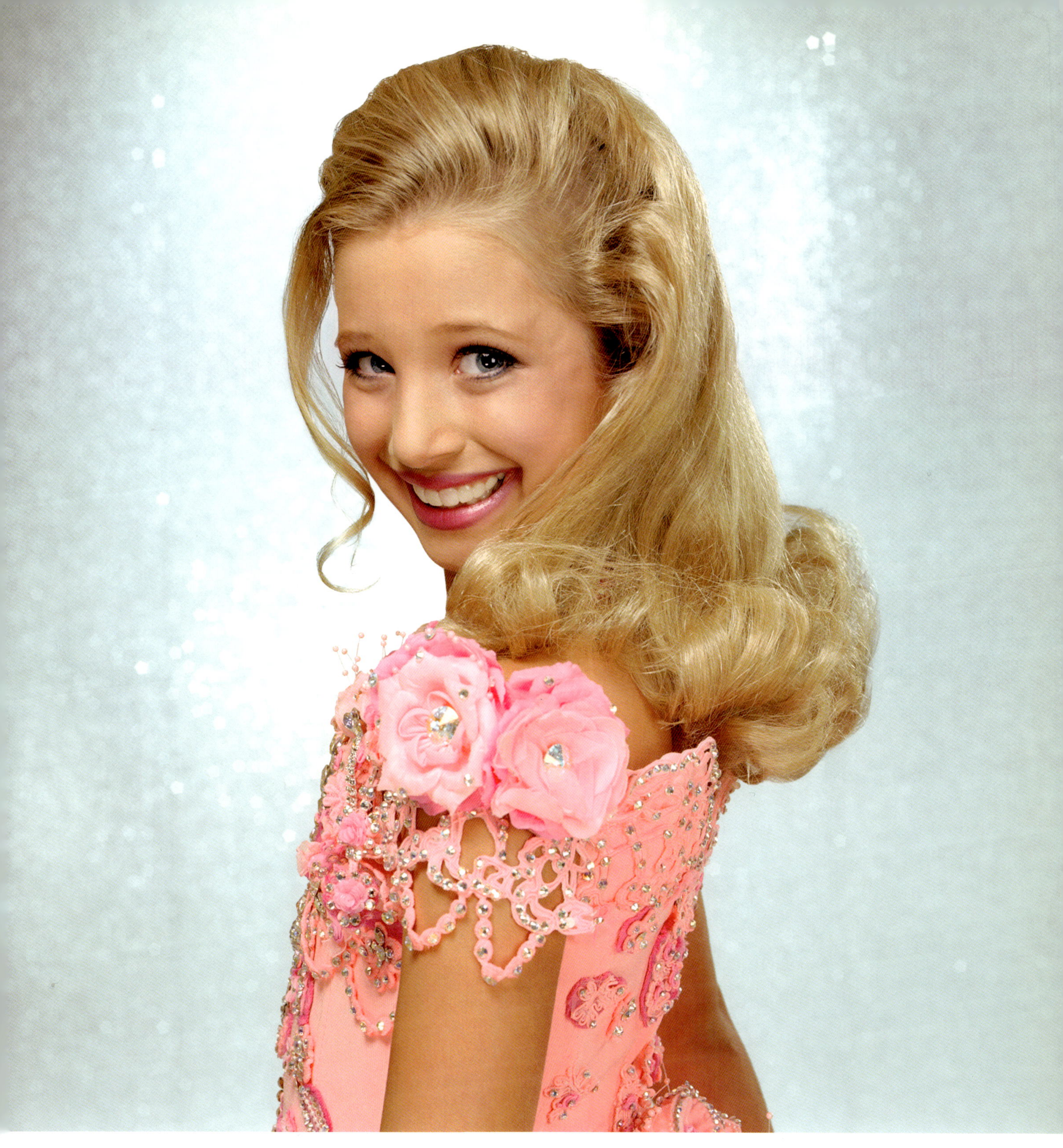

Age 8 × Austin, Texas × 2005

Sara

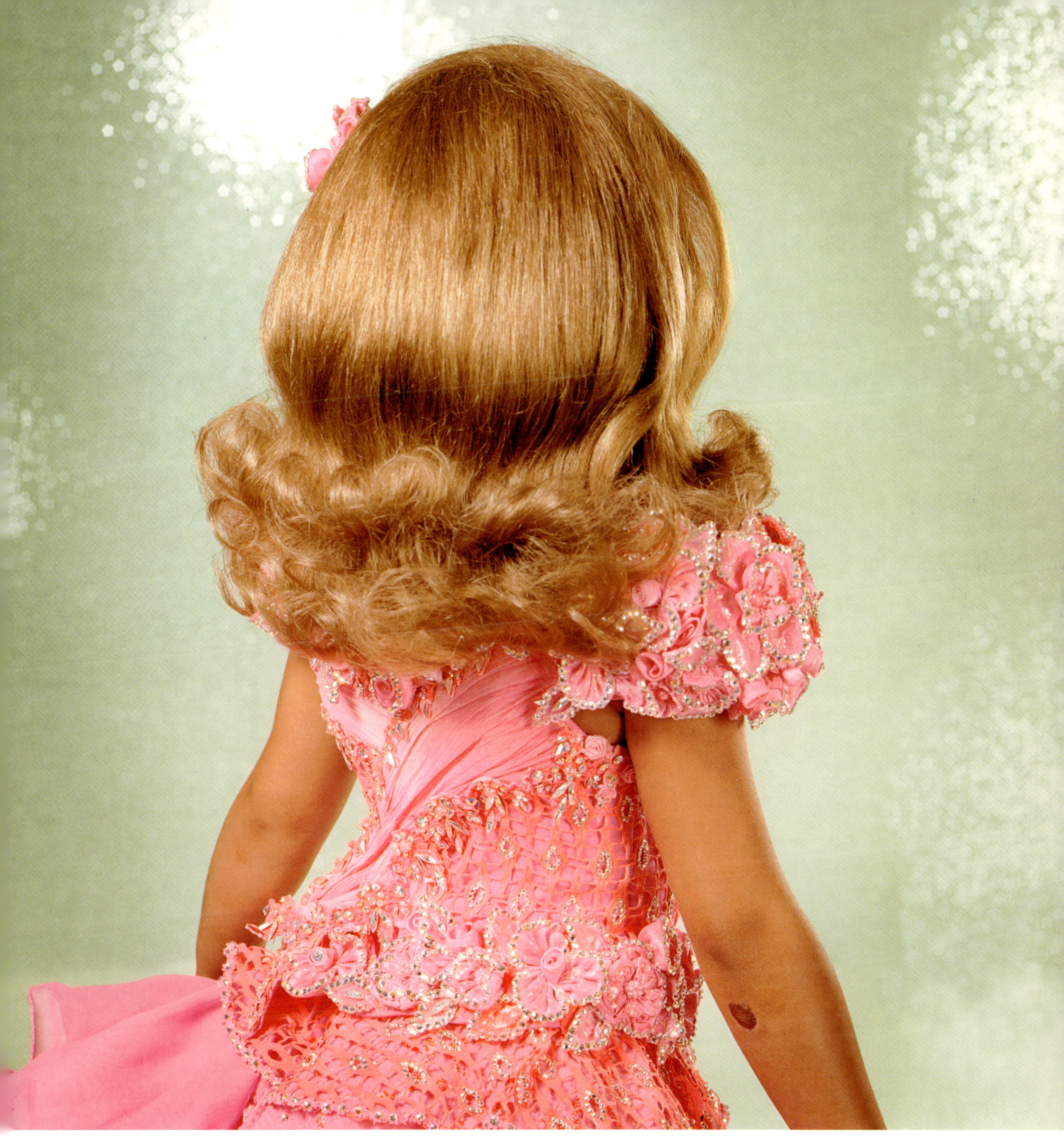

Age 5 × Las Vegas, Nevada × 2006

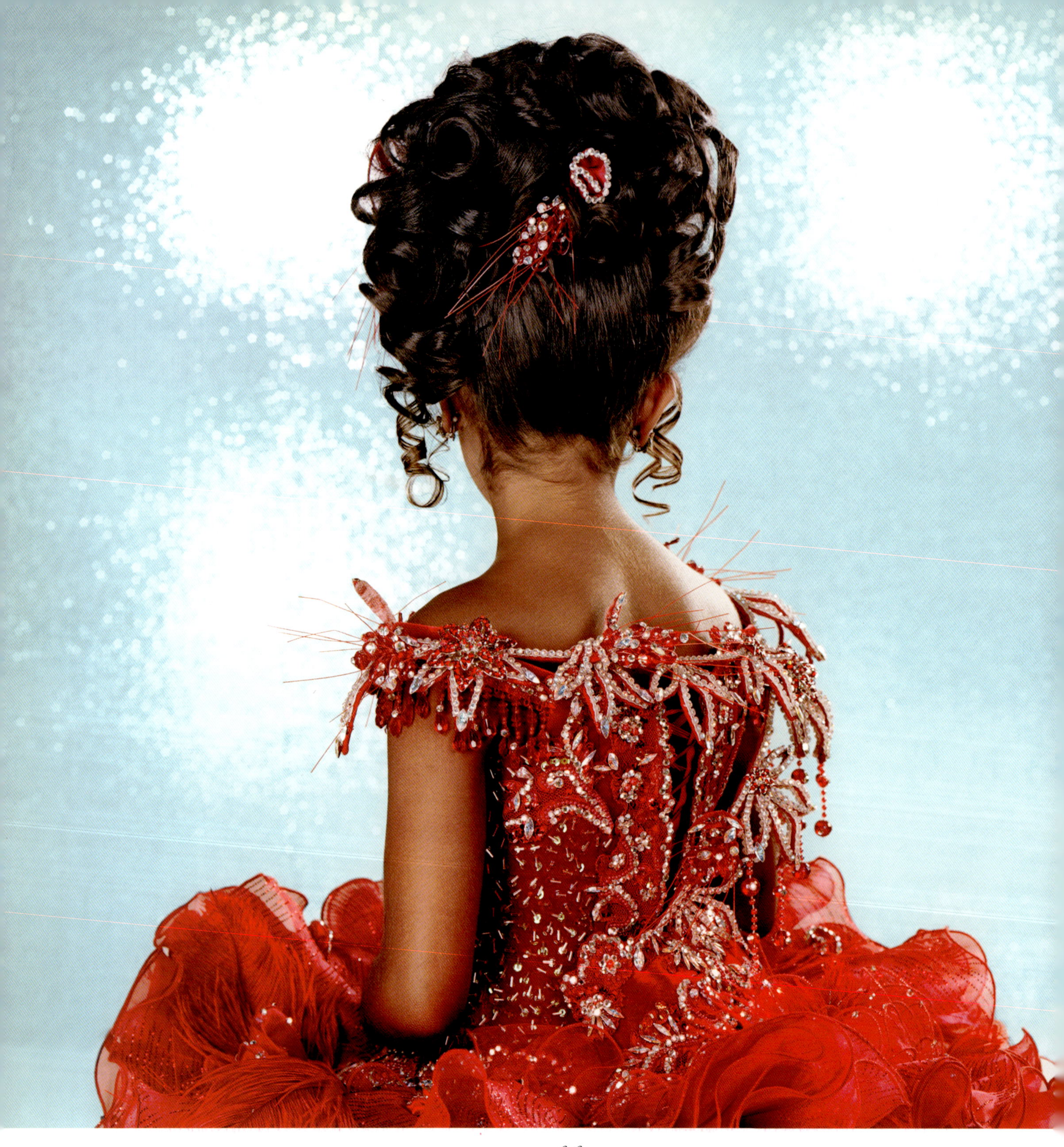

Ashley

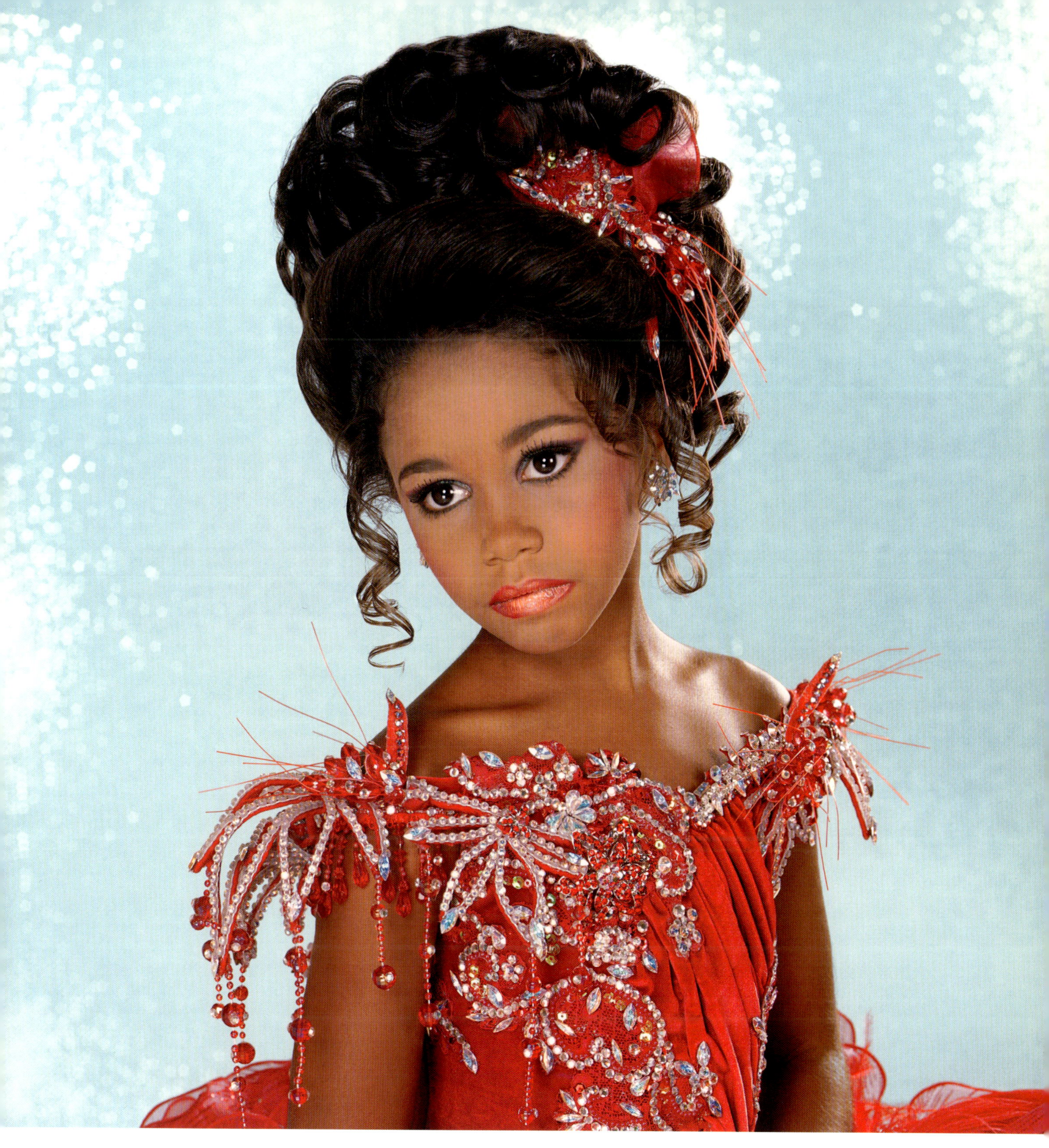

Age 8 × Nashville, Tennessee × 2008

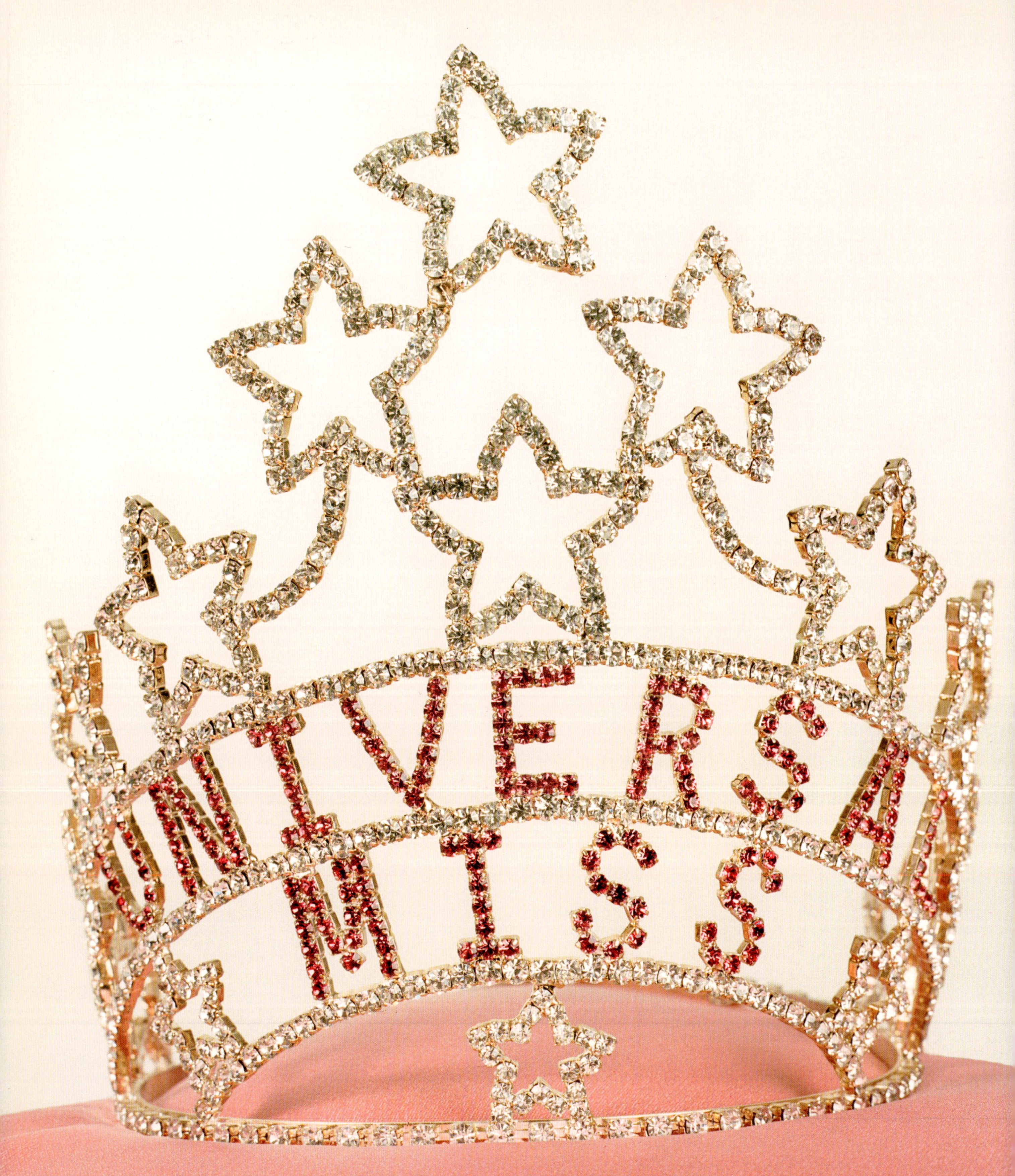
UNIVERSA
MISS

Modeling

Jacklyn

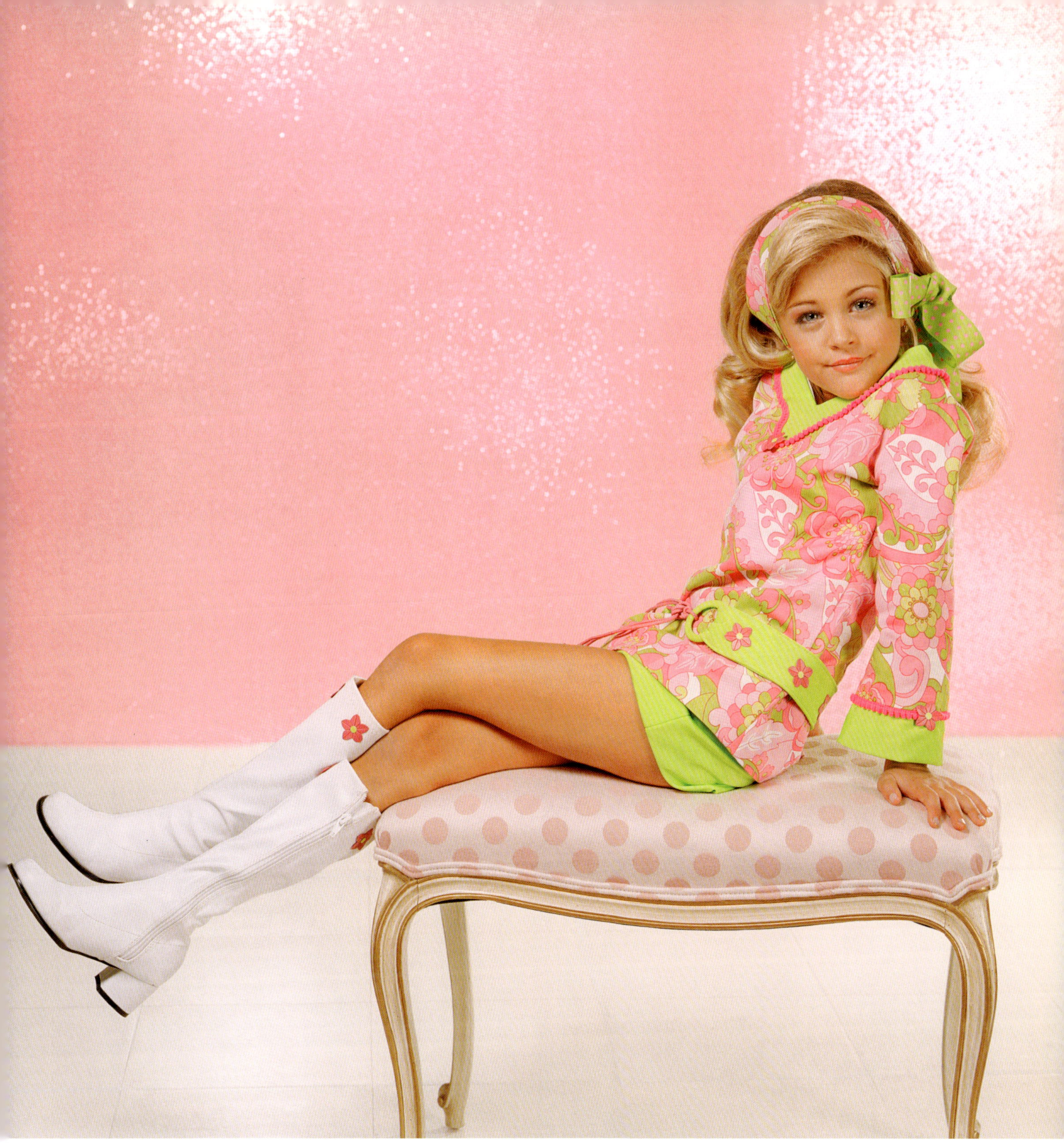

Age 7 × Las Vegas, Nevada × 2006

Stephanie

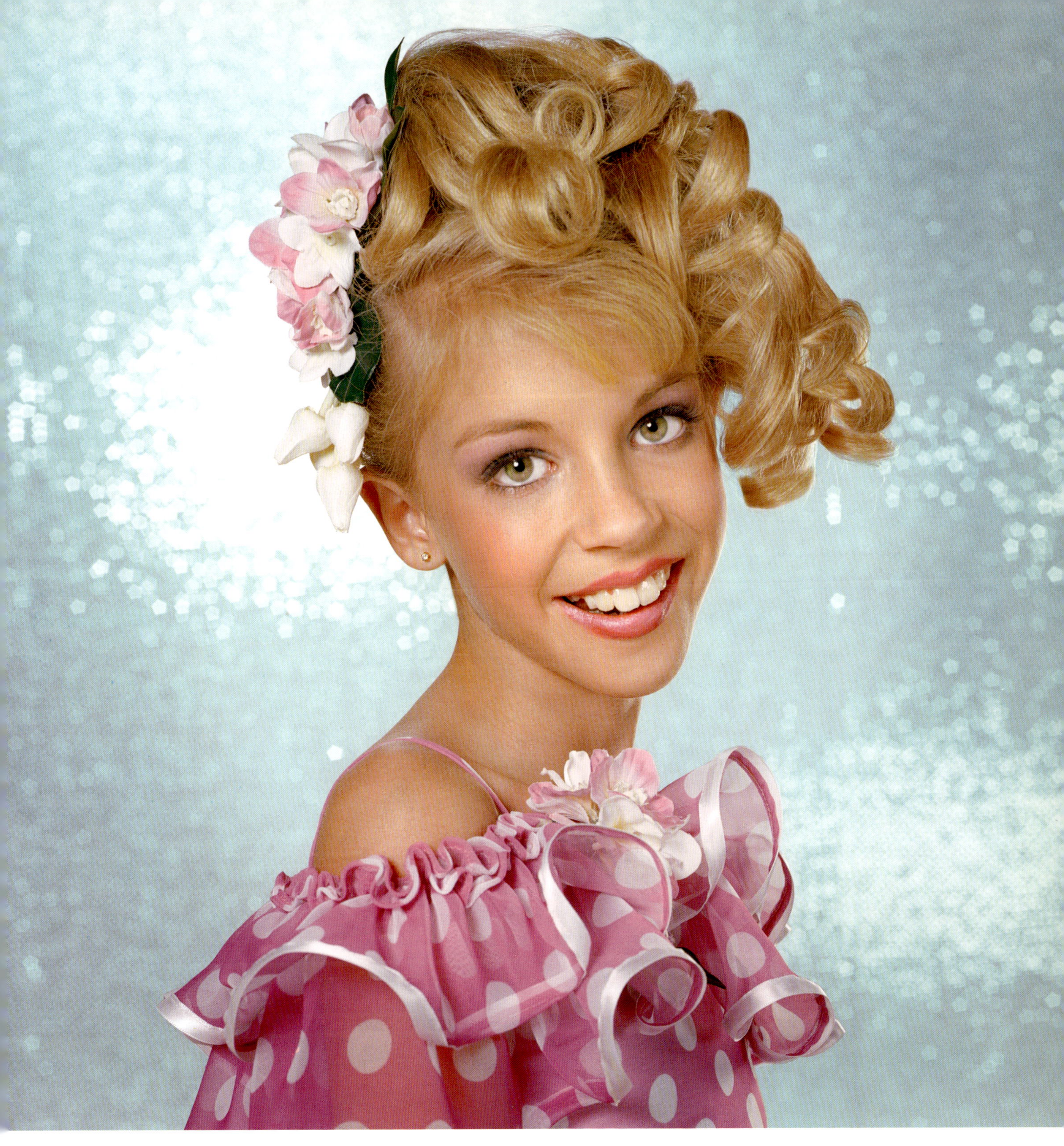

Age 9 ✕ Santa Ana, California ✕ 2005

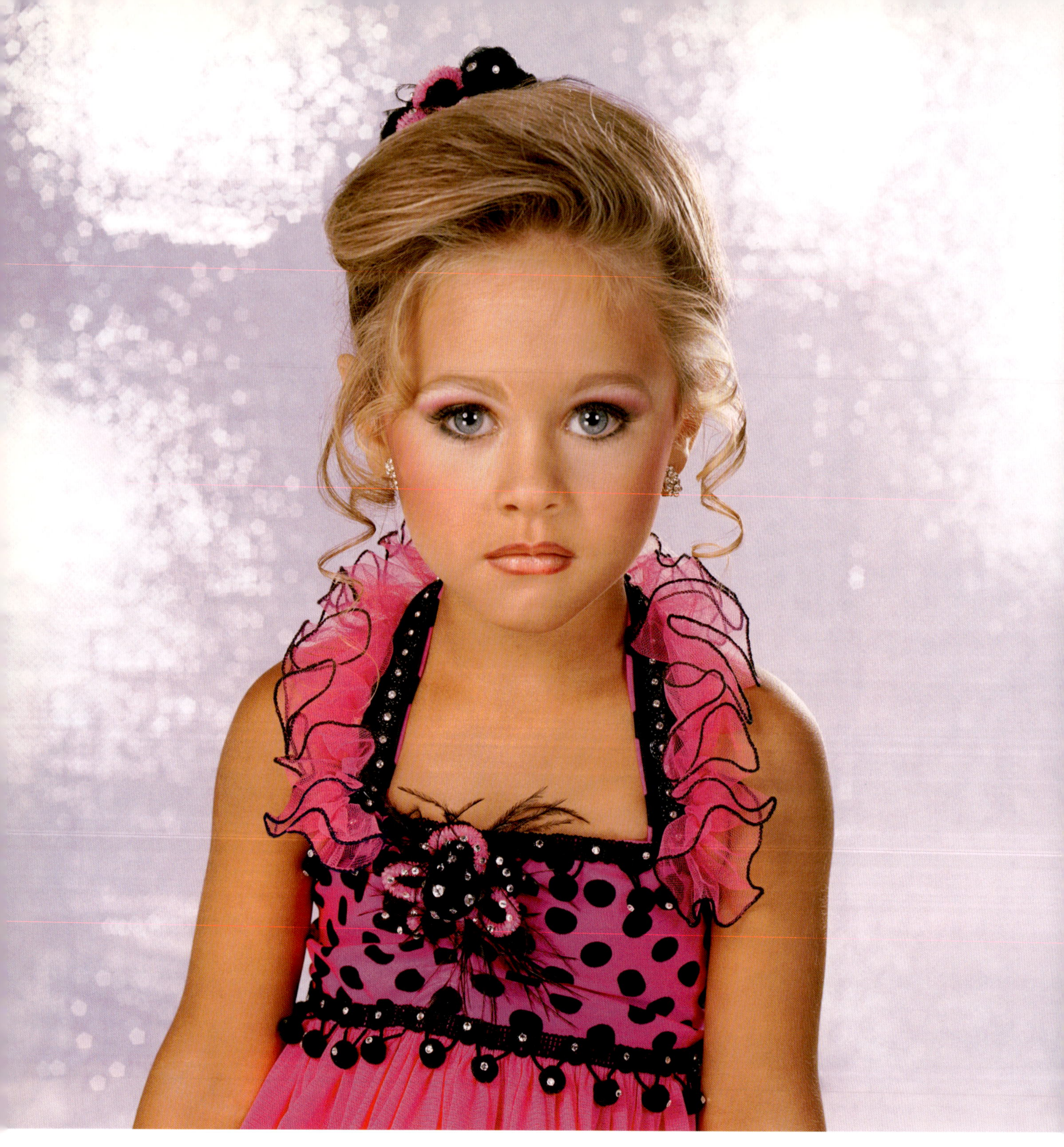

Destiny

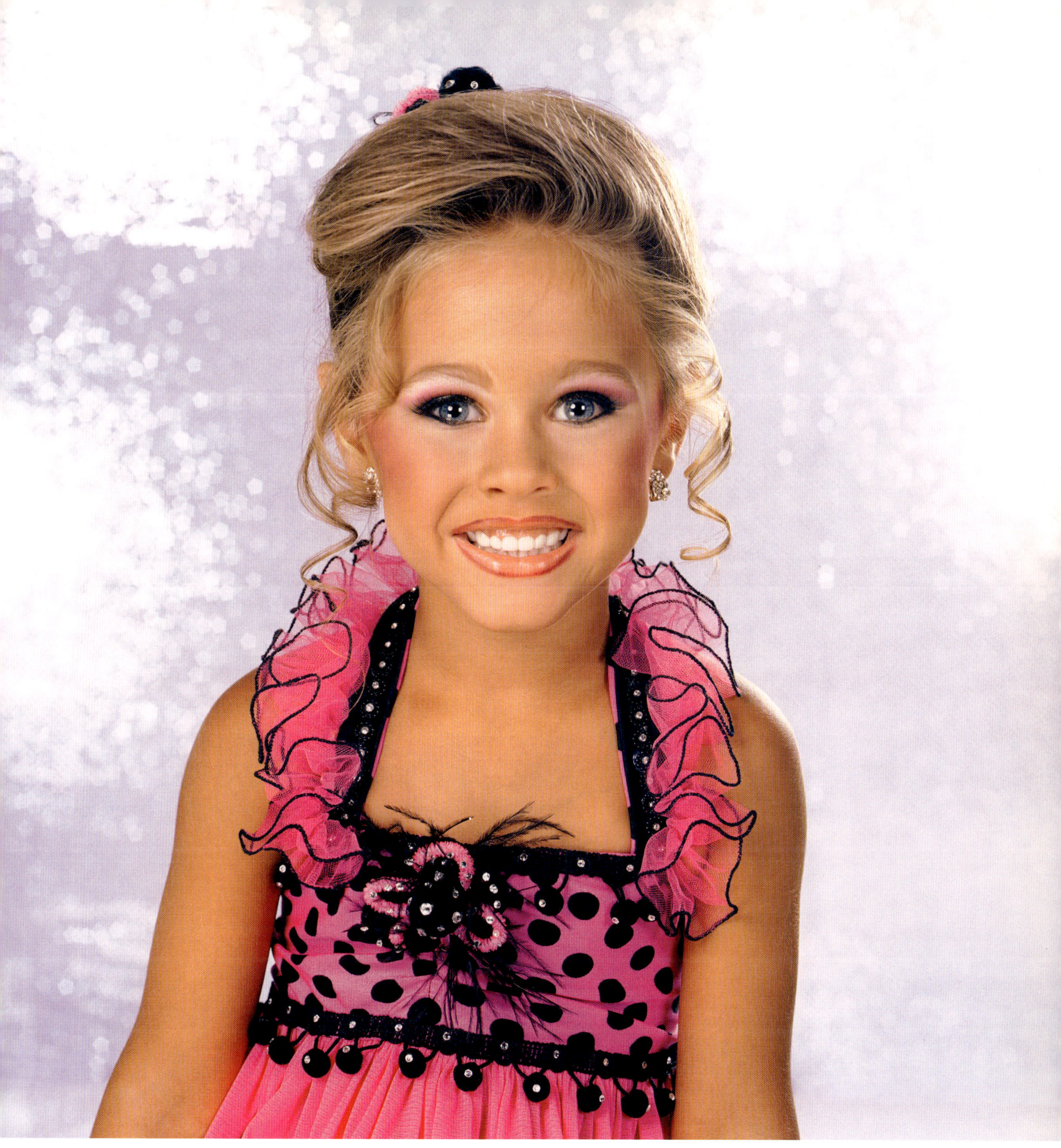

Age 5 × Nashville, Tennessee × 2008

Alex

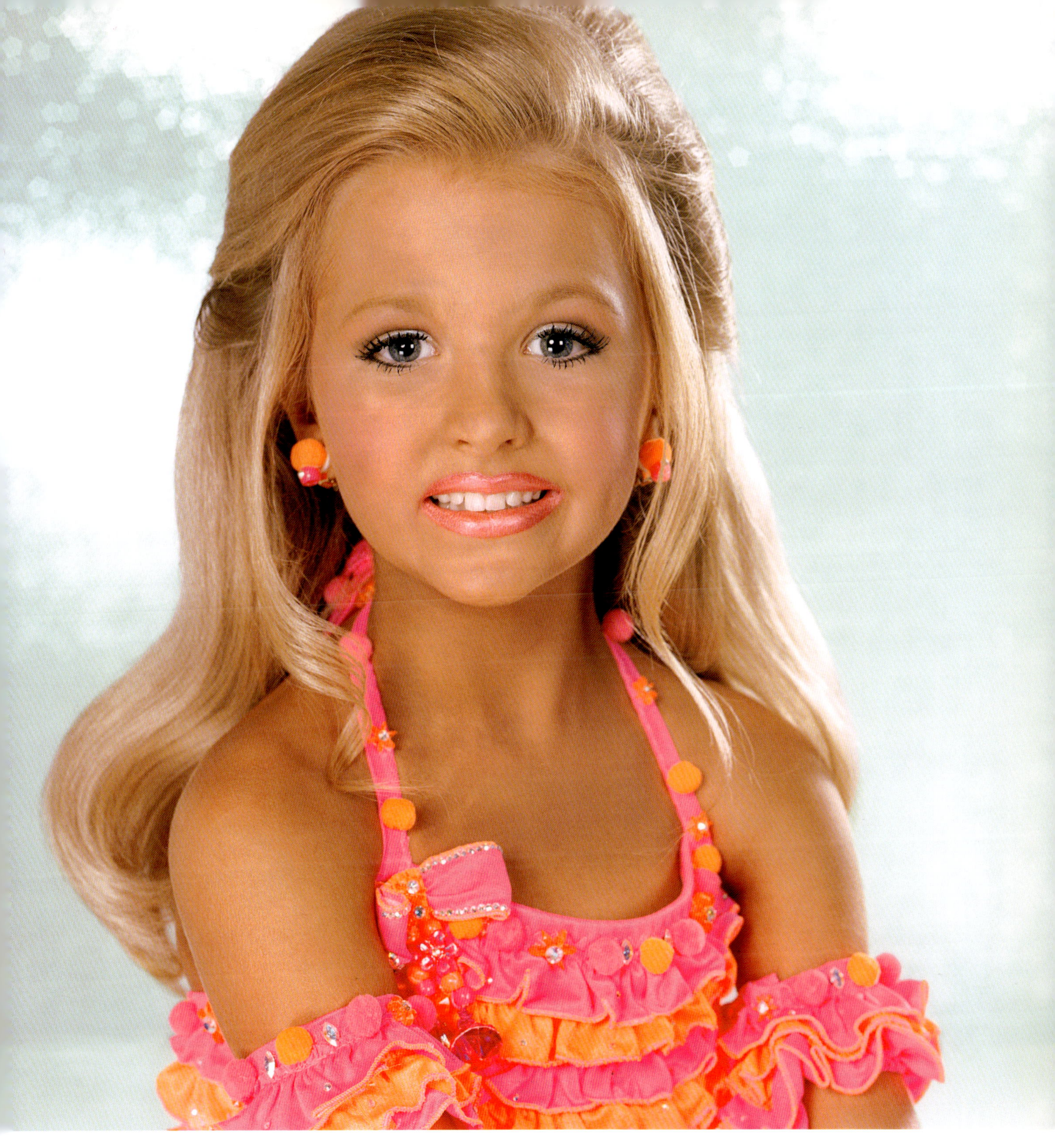

Age 7 ✶ Nashville, Tennessee ✶ 2008

Sara

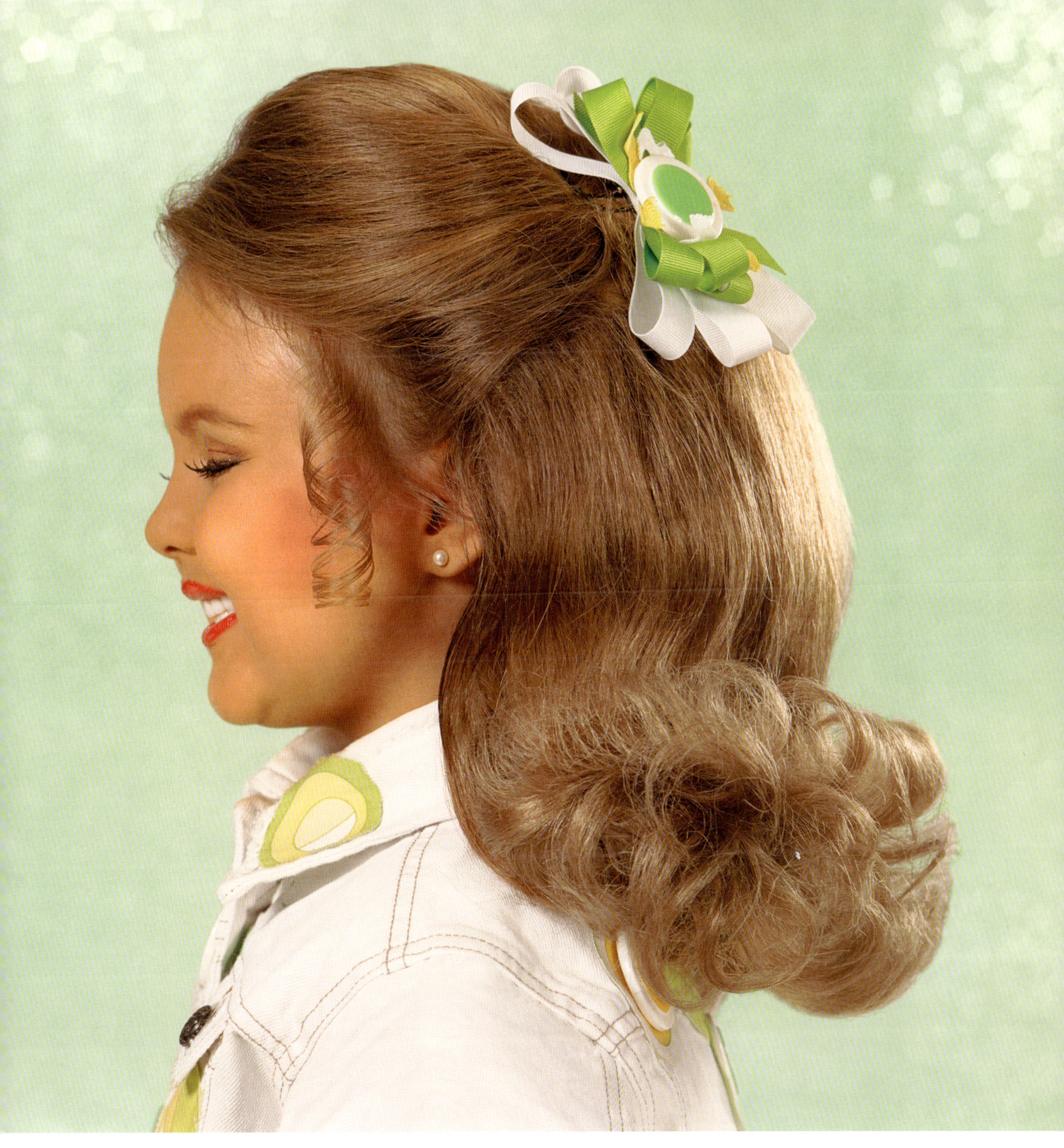

Age 5 × Las Vegas, Nevada × 2006

Katy

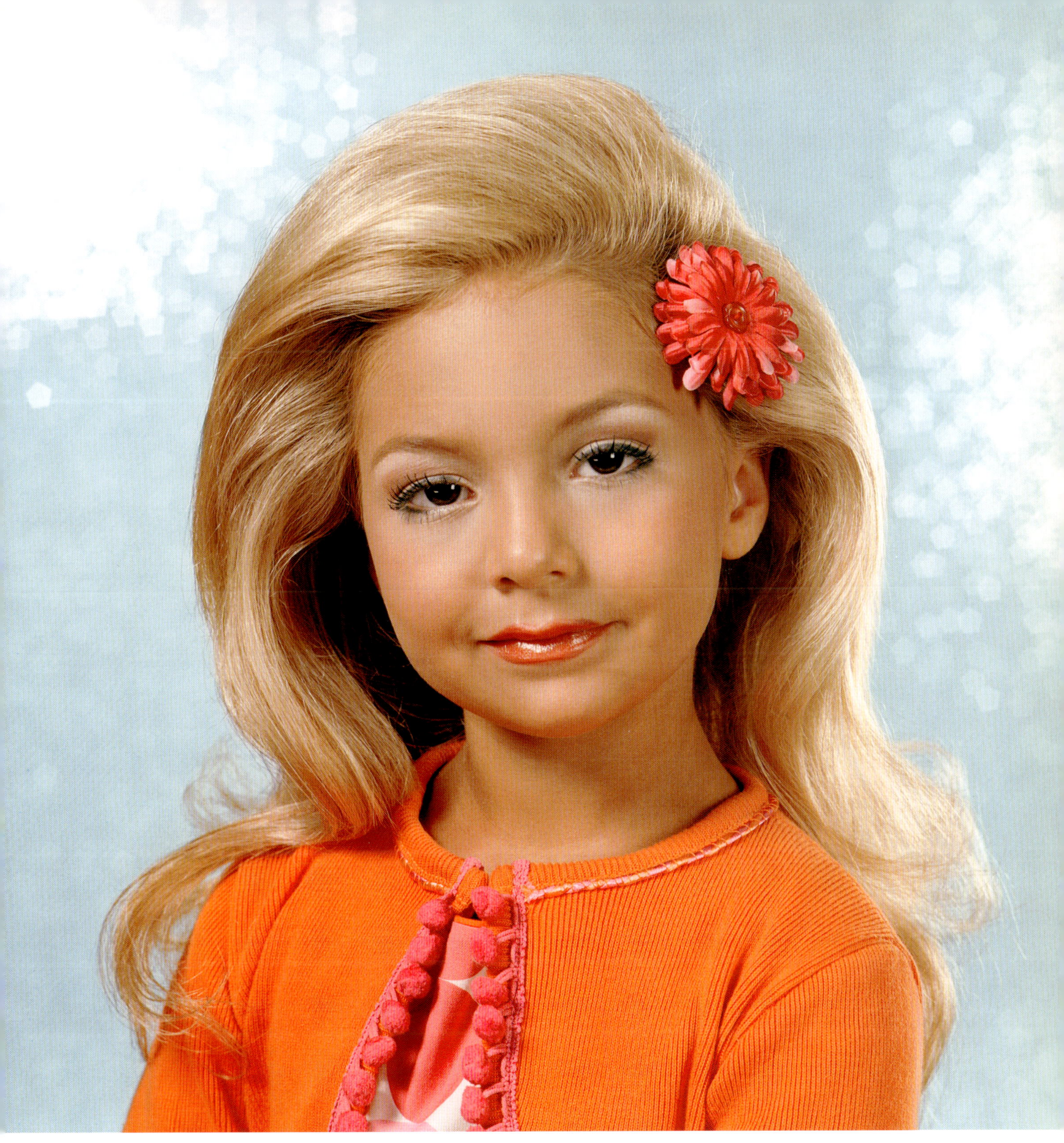

Age 5 × Las Vegas, Nevada × 2006

Savanha

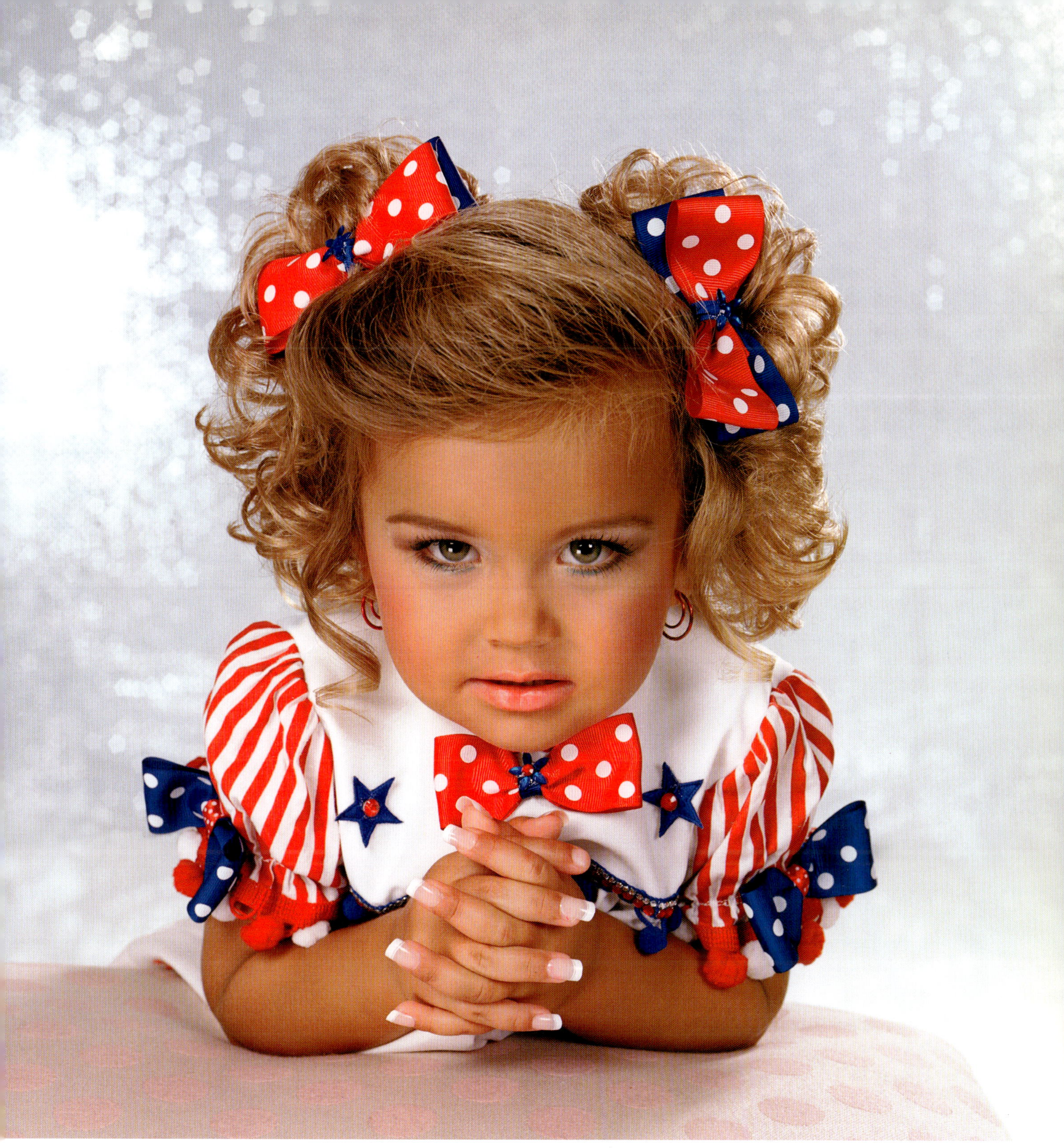

Age 2 × Nashville, Tennessee × 2008

Danica

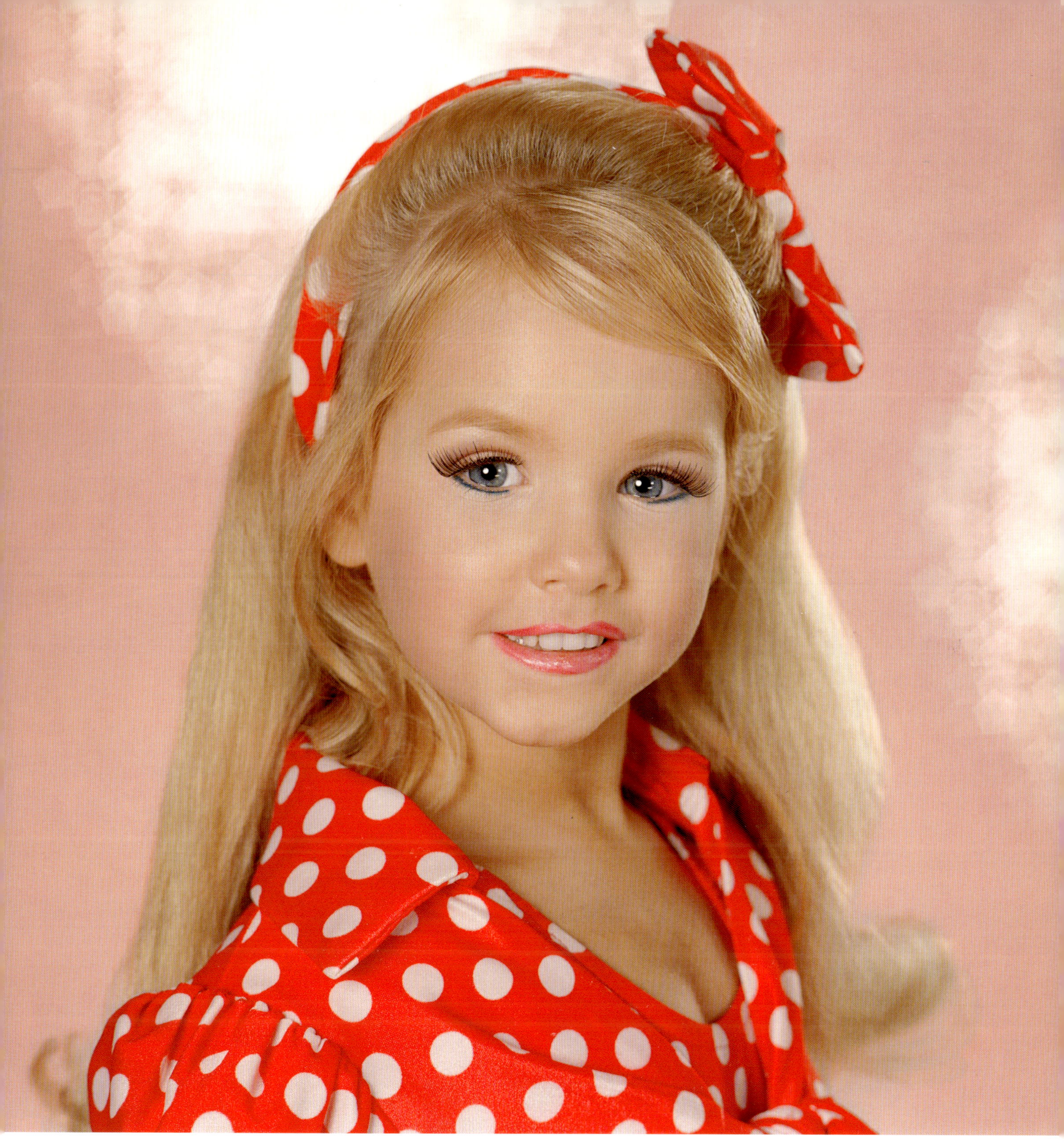

Age 5 × Santa Ana, California × 2005

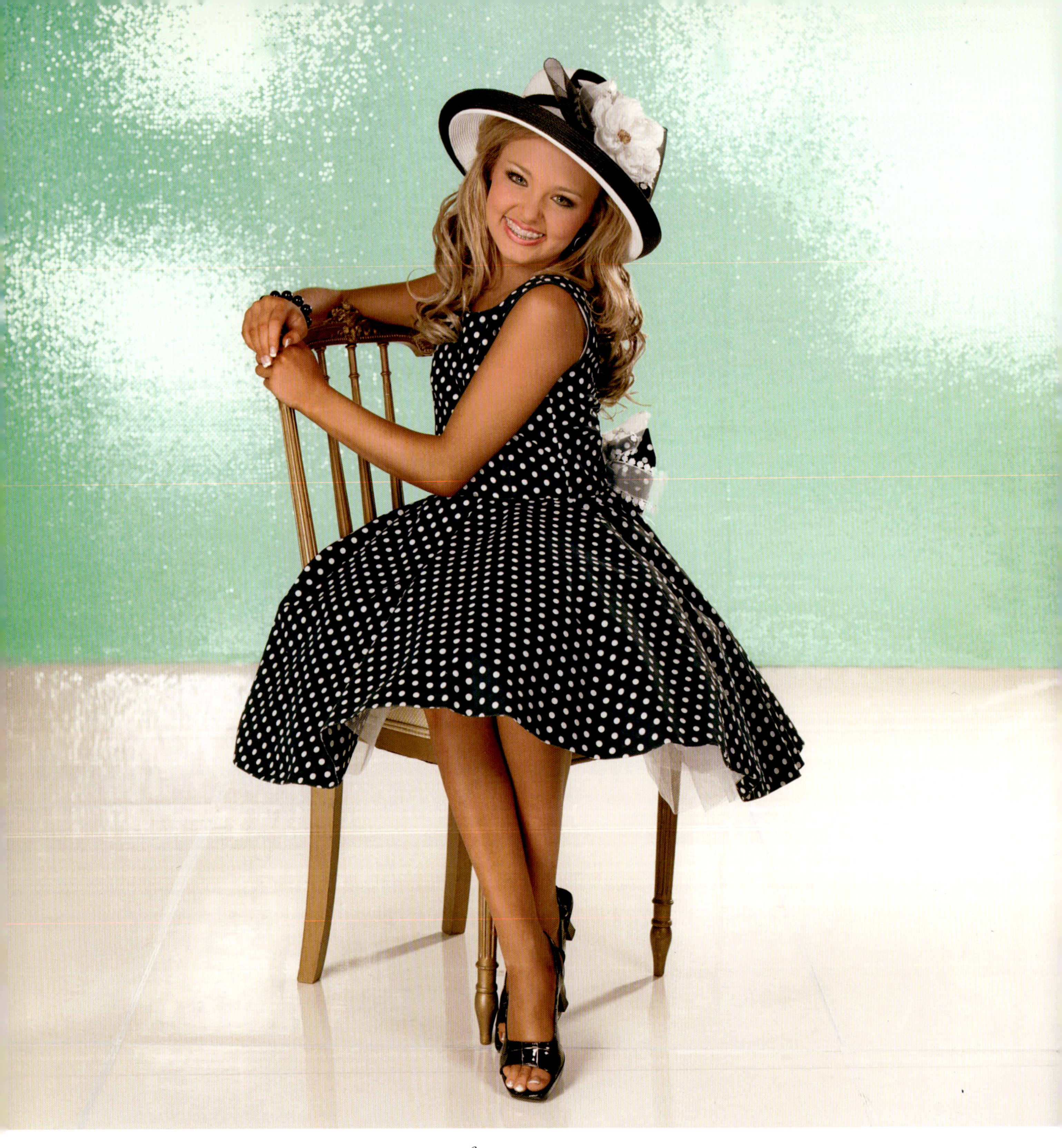

Mary Ashton × Age 9 × Nashville, Tennessee × 2008

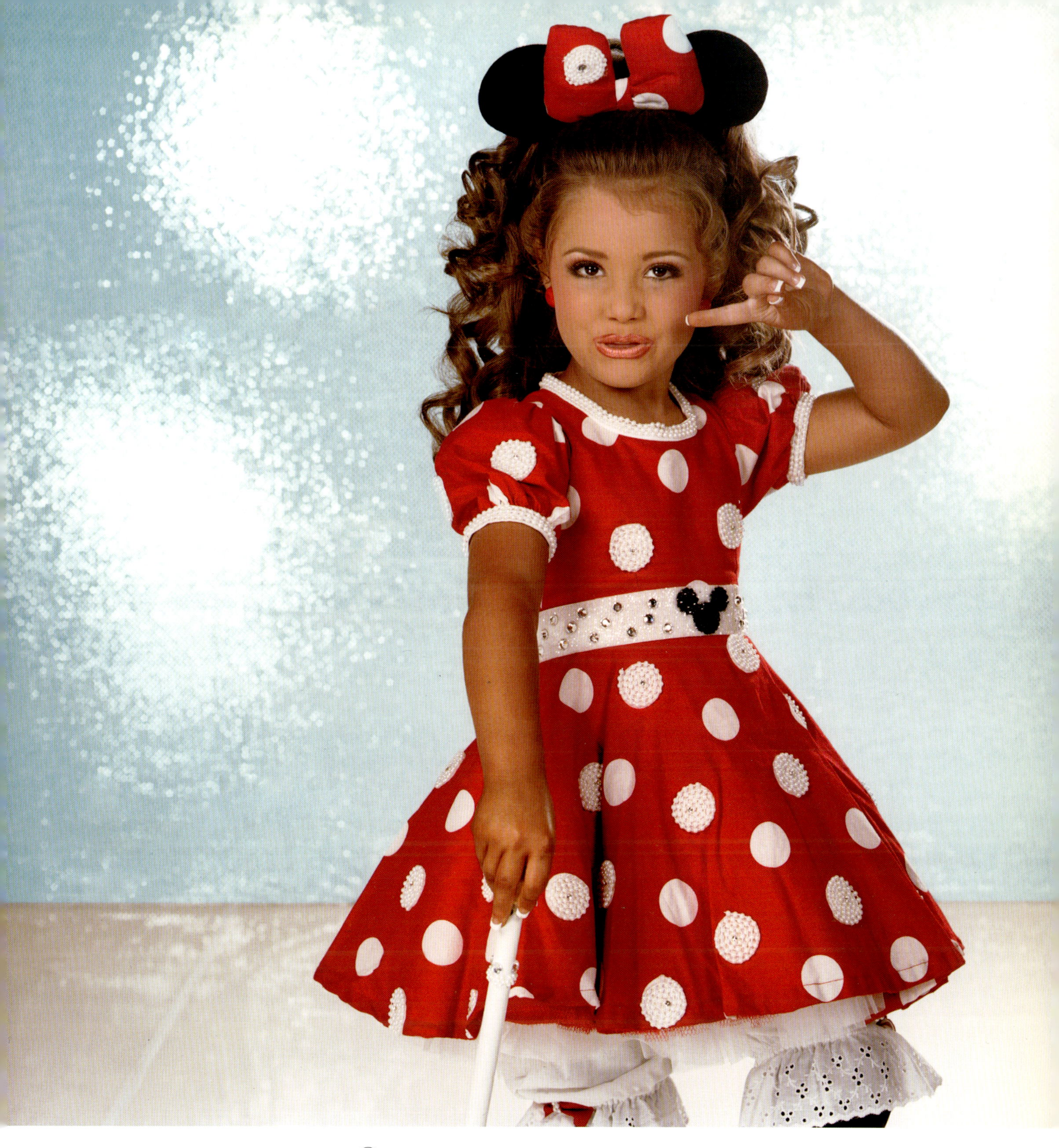

Tatum × Age 5 × Nashville, Tennessee × 2008

Amiaya

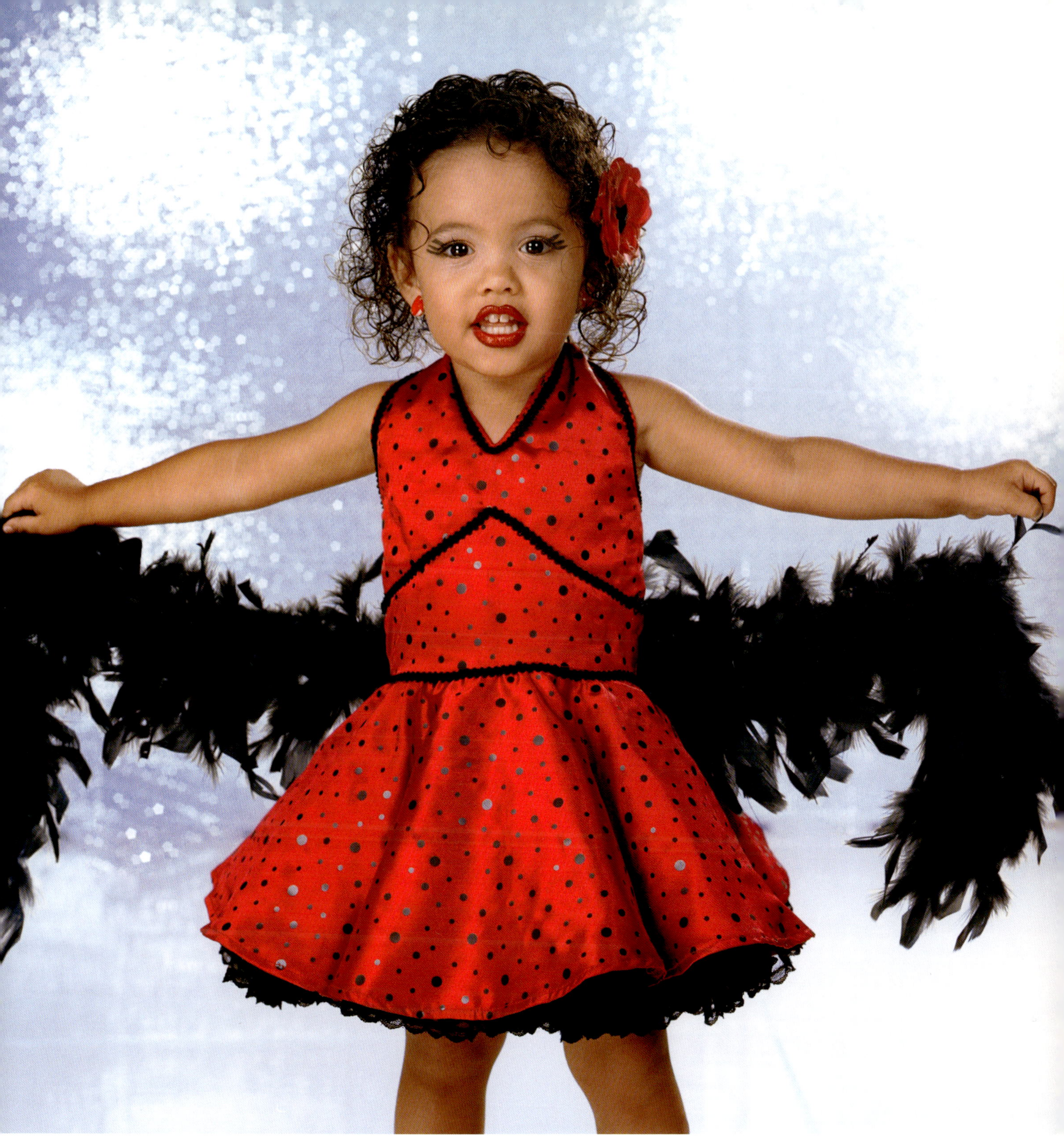

Age 2 ✶ Nashville, Tennessee ✶ 2008

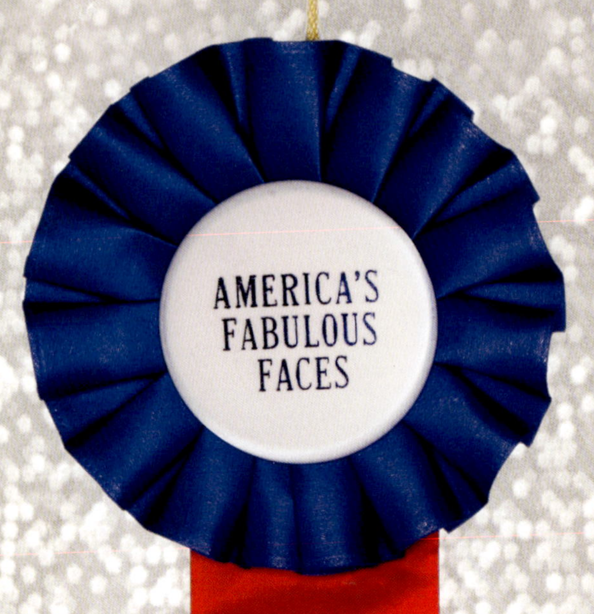
AMERICA'S
FABULOUS
FACES
BEST
HAIR
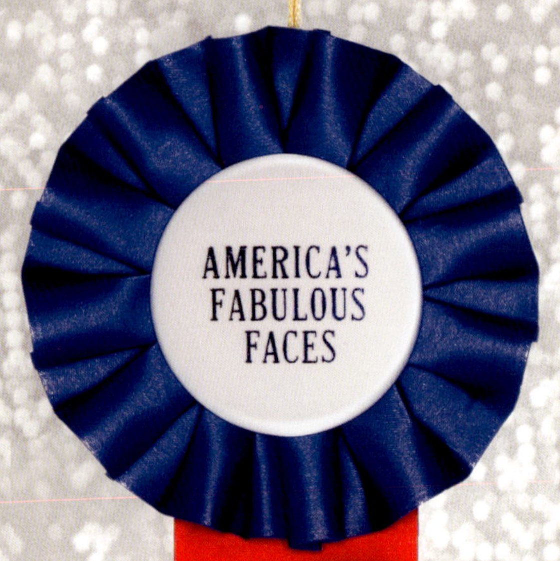
AMERICA'S
FABULOUS
FACES
BEST
EYES

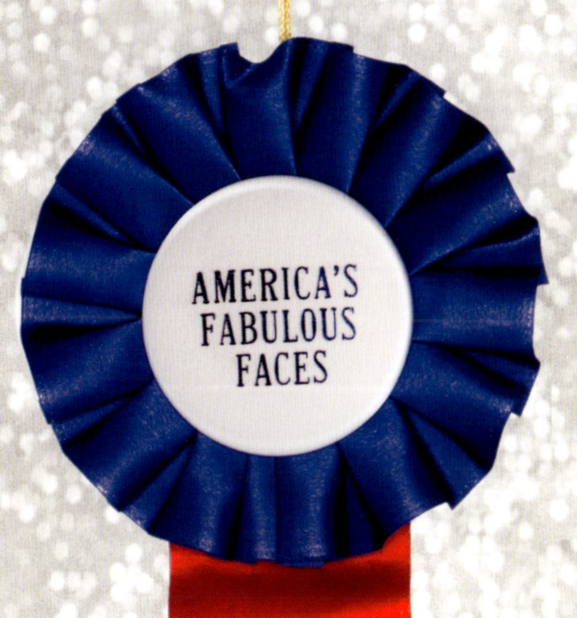
AMERICA'S
FABULOUS
FACES
BEST
SMILE

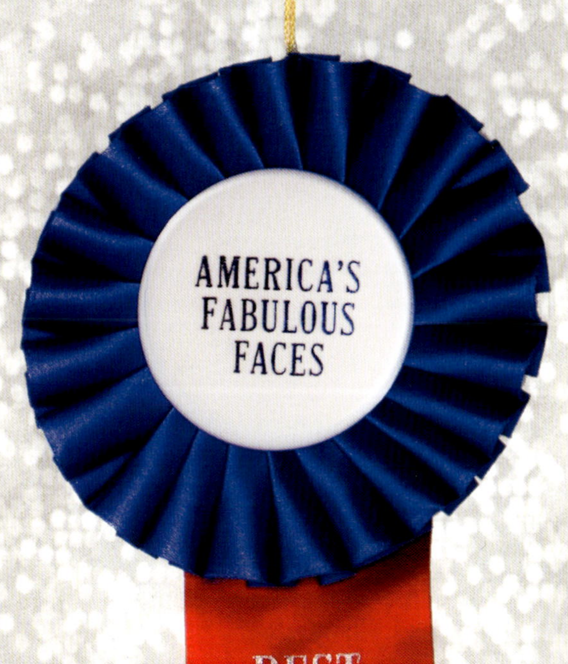
AMERICA'S
FABULOUS
FACES
BEST
PERSONALITY

Lexi

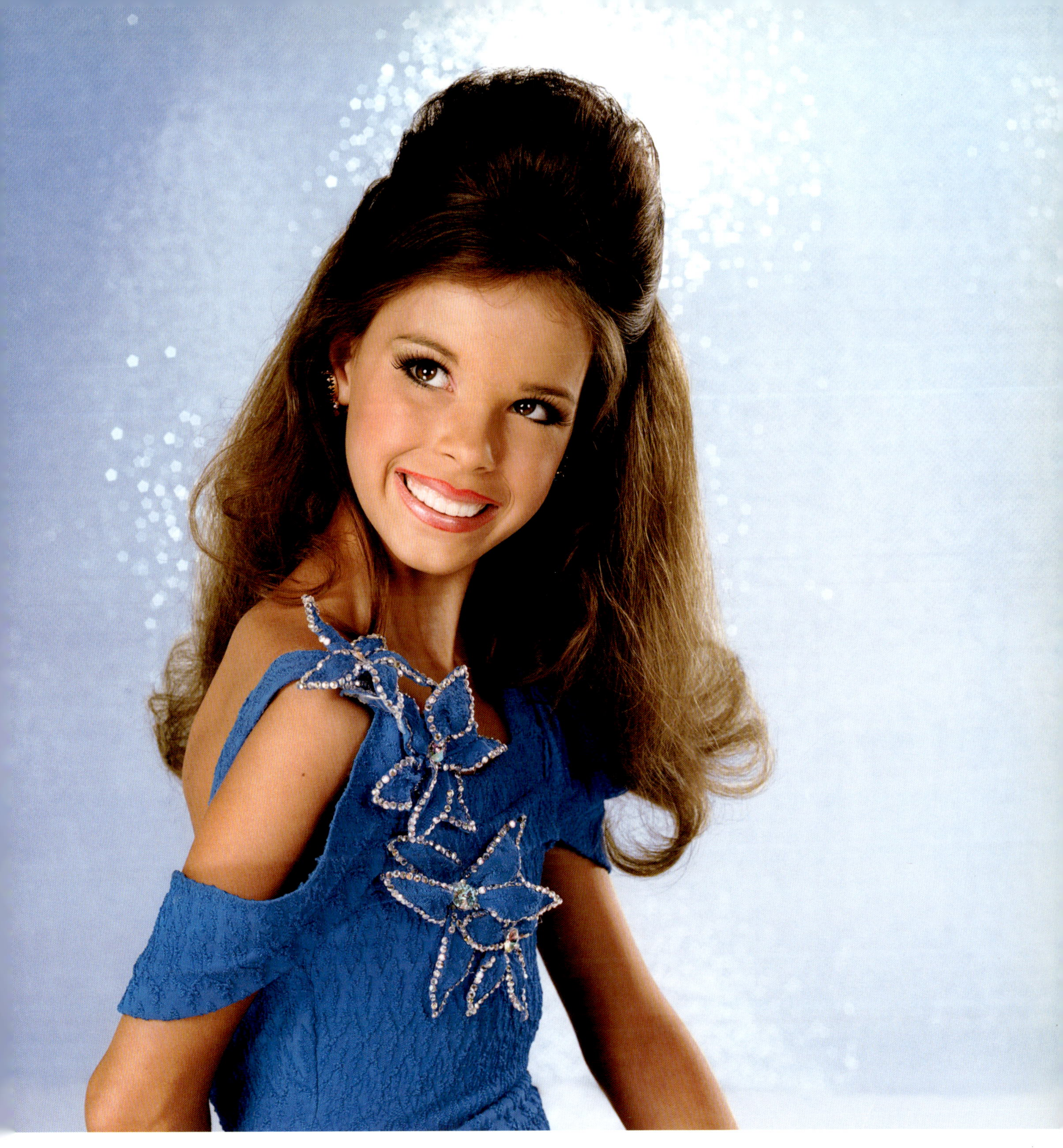

Age 9 ✶ Nashville, Tennessee ✶ 2008

Mary Ashton

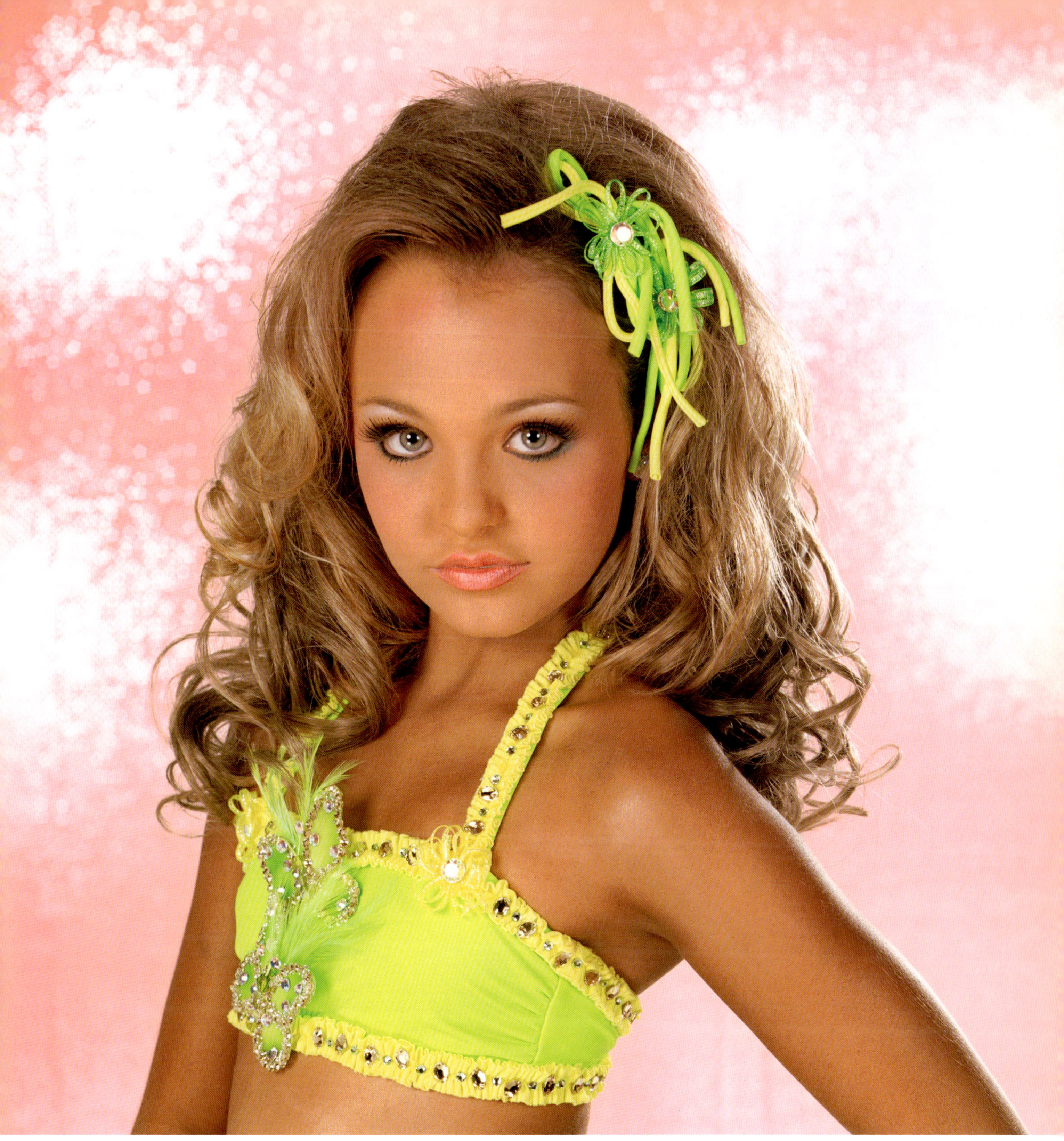

Age 9 × Nashville, Tennessee × 2008

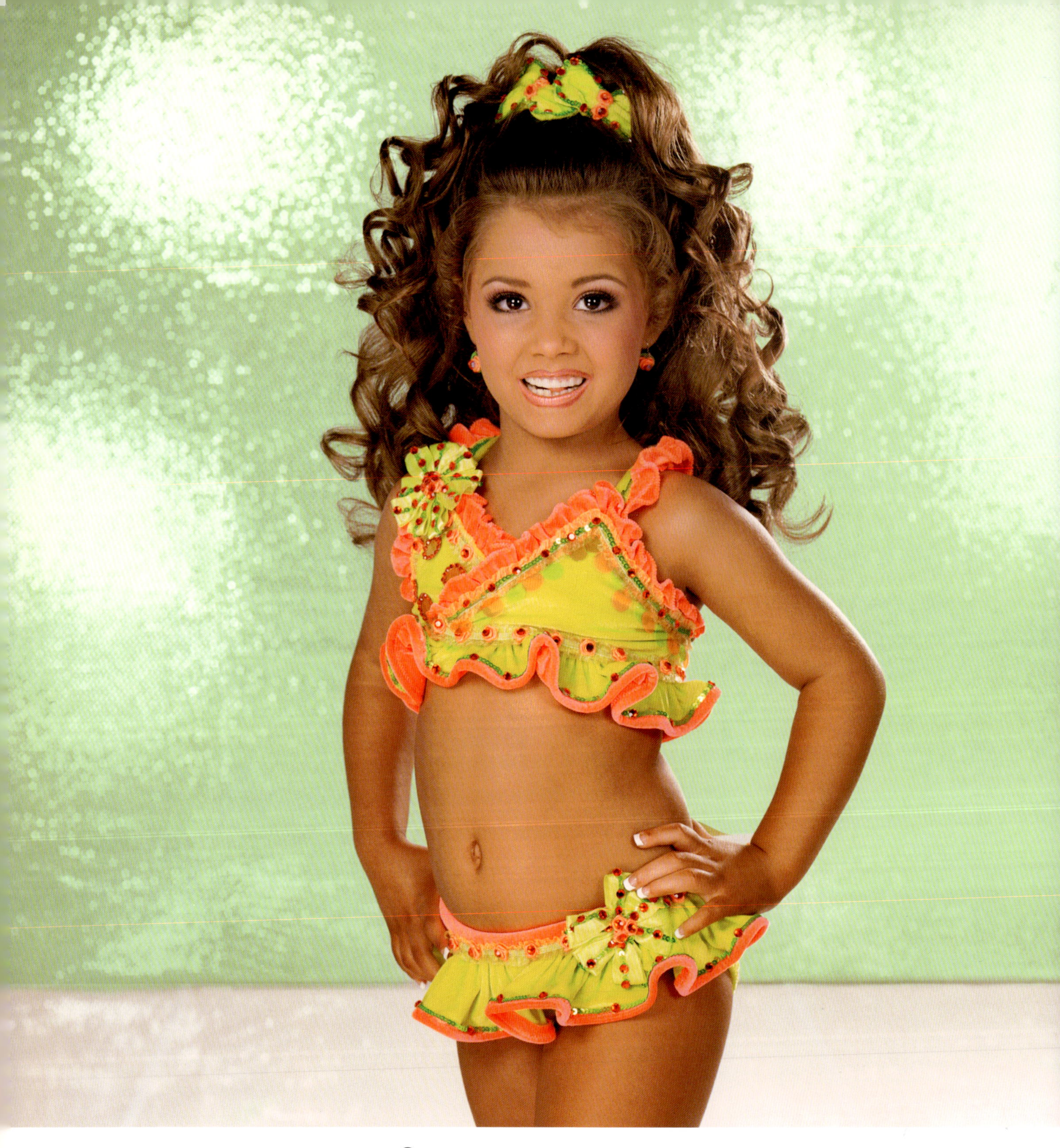

Tatum × Age 5 × Nashville, Tennessee × 2008

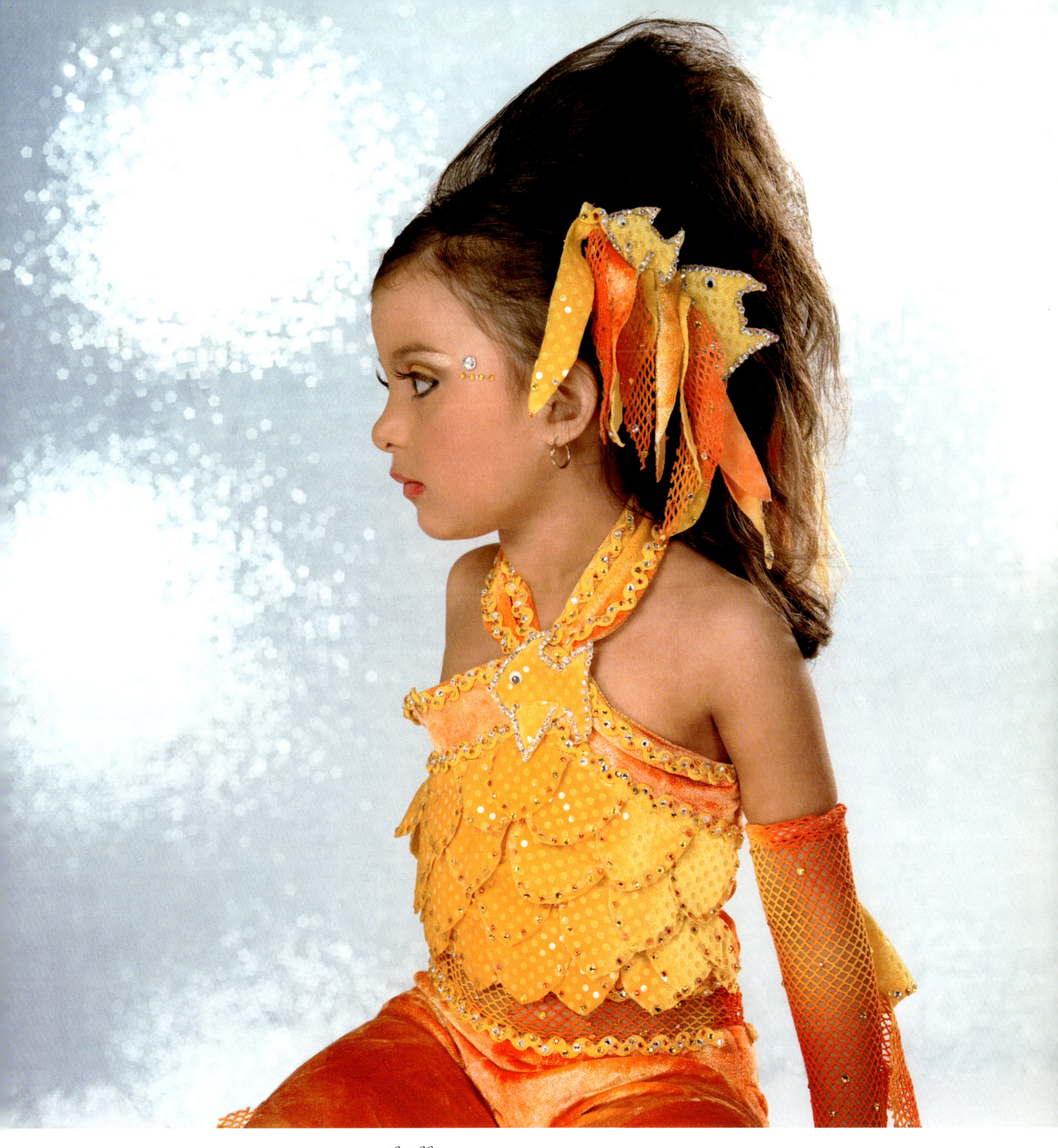

Isabella × Age 3 × Nashville, Tennessee × 2008

Lauren

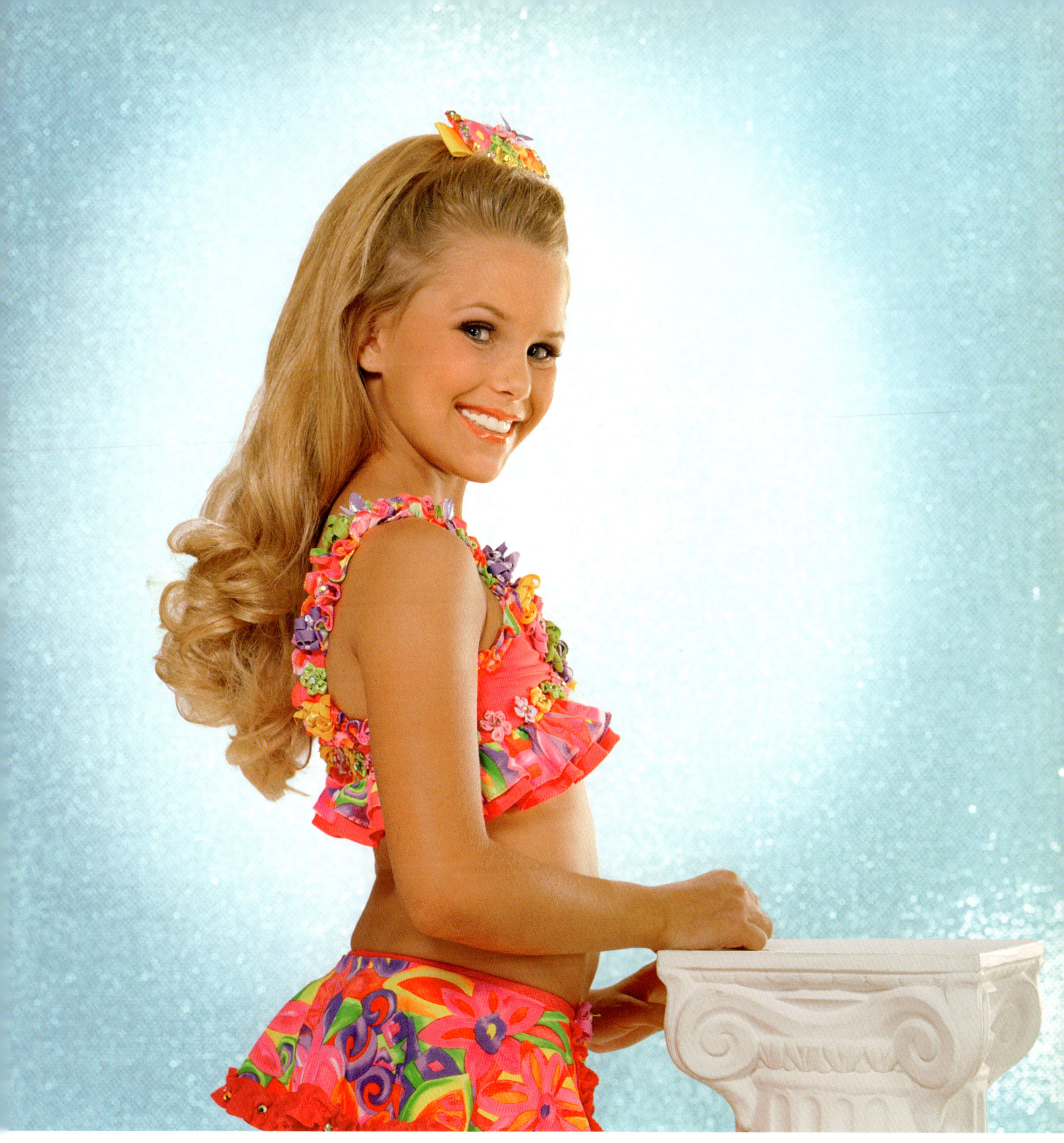

Age 10 × Santa Ana, California × 2005

Kasinda

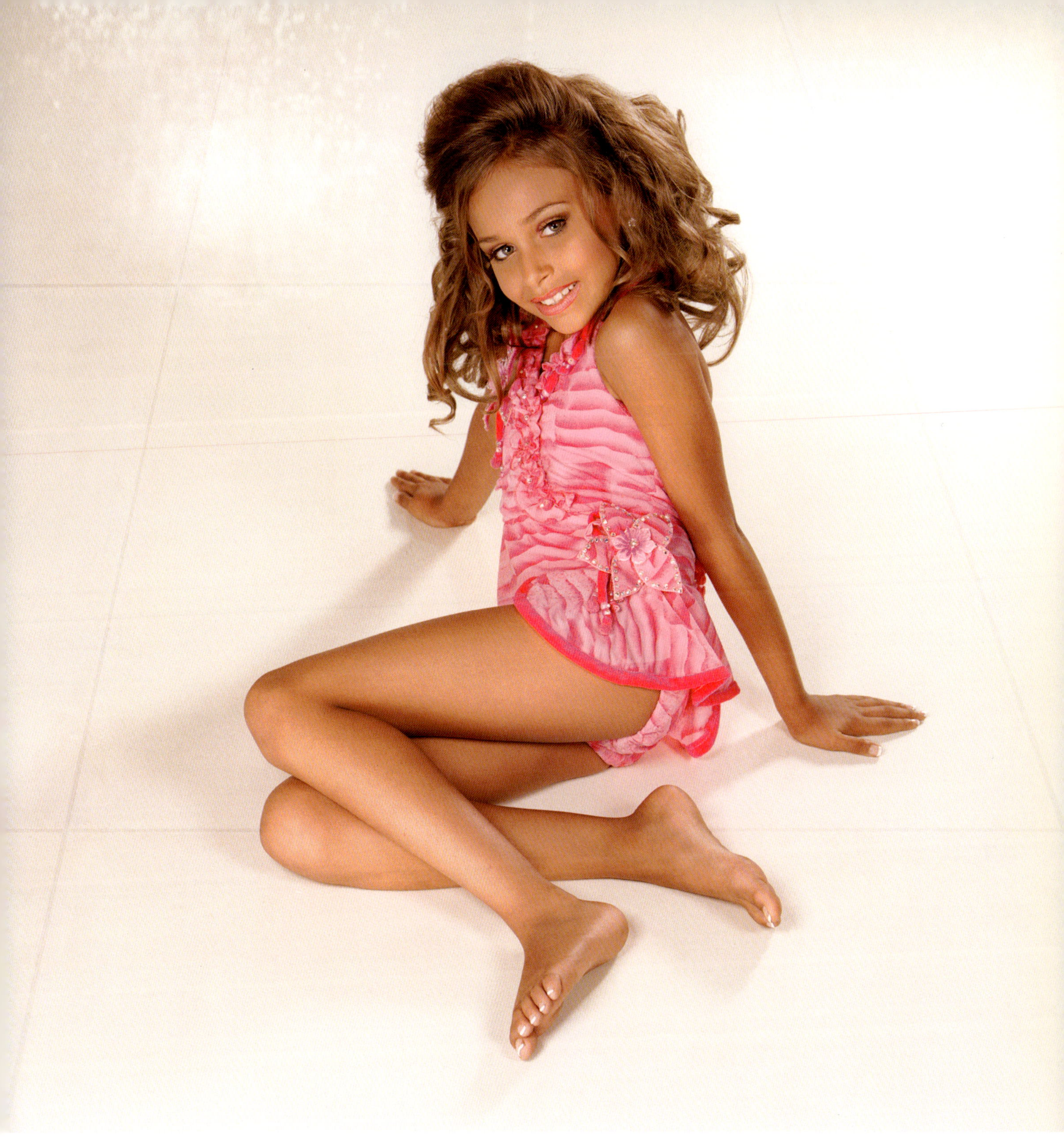

Age 8 ✕ Nashville, Tennessee ✕ 2008

Carley

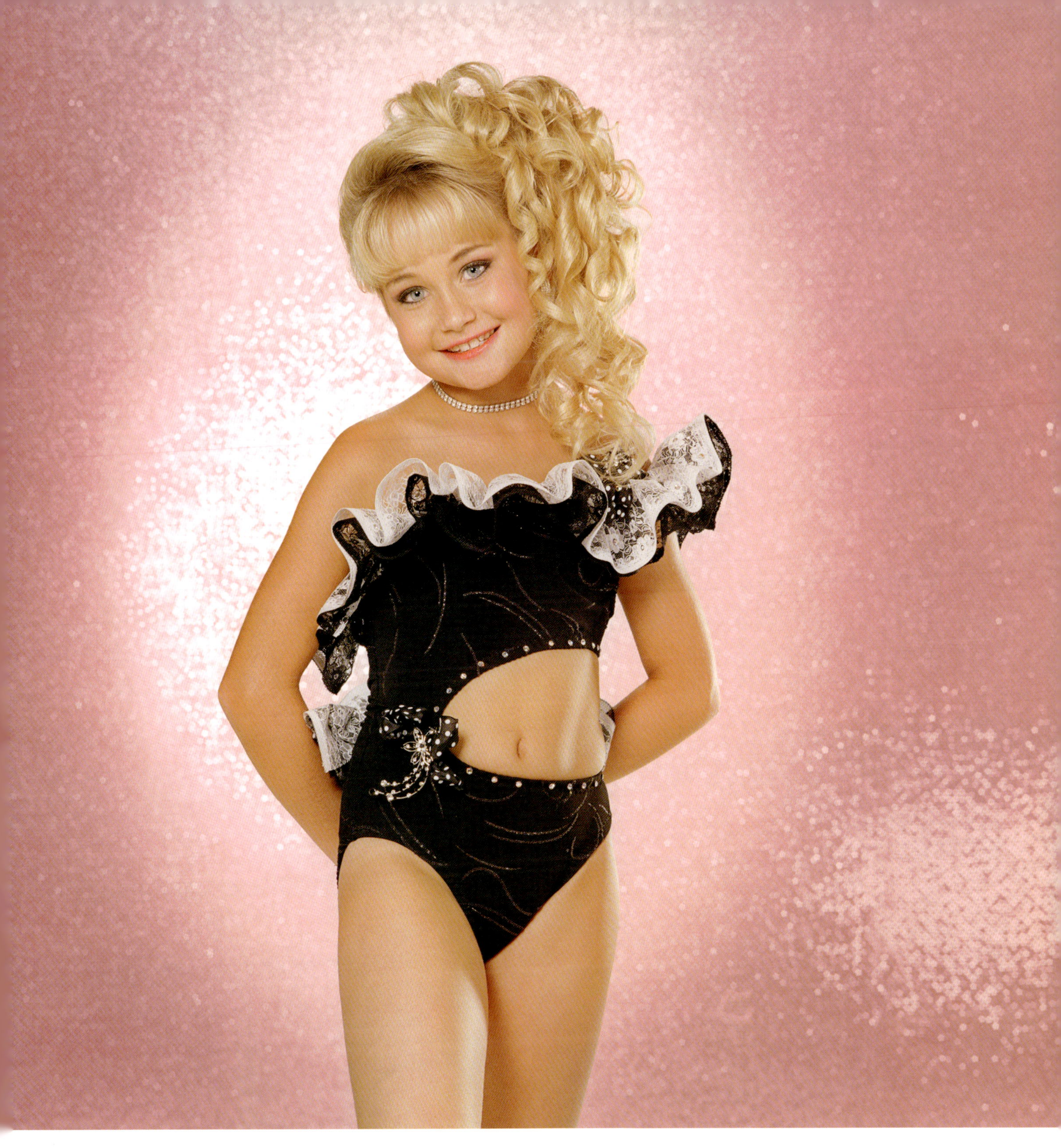

Age 9 × Santa Ana, California × 2005

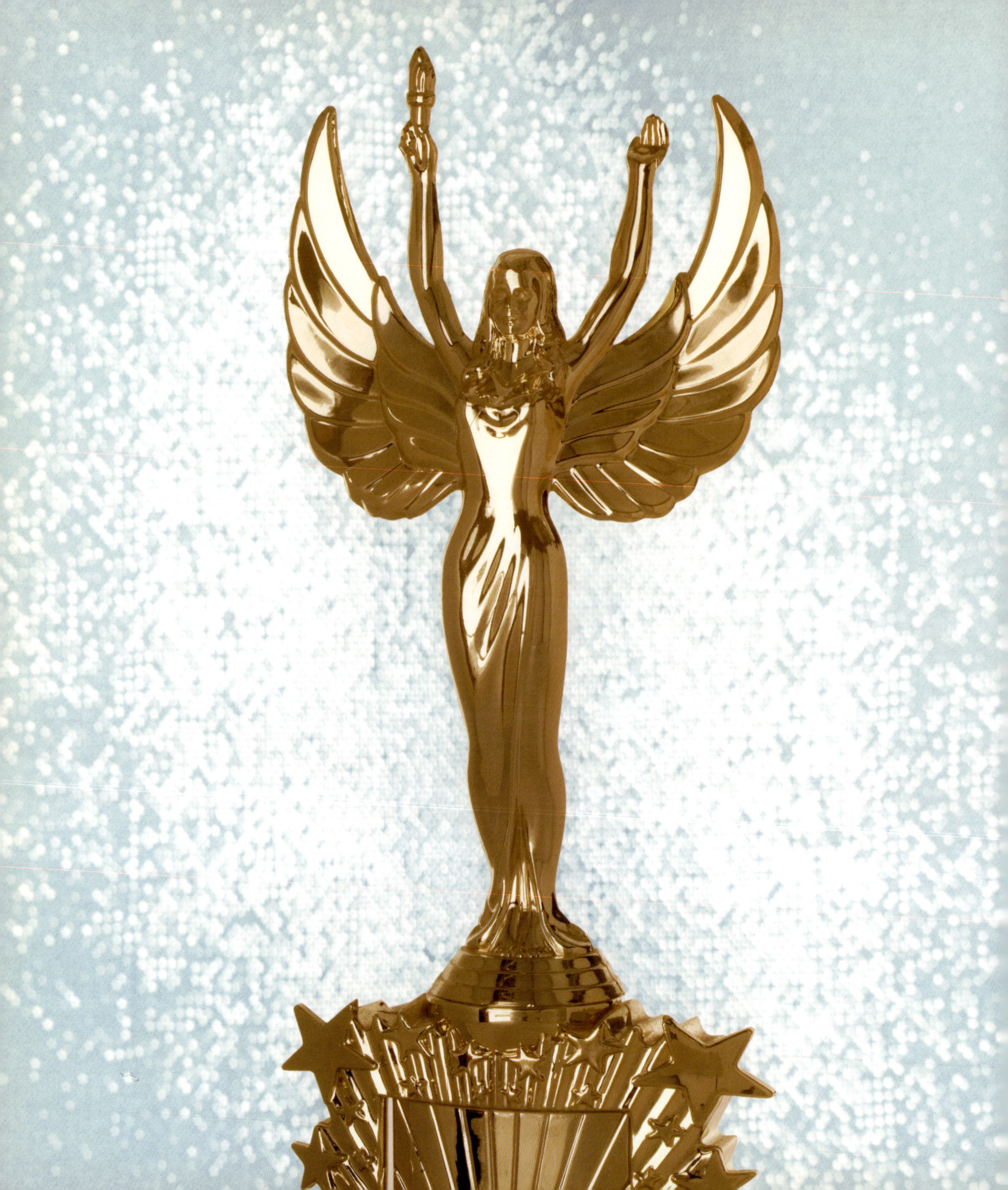

Western Wear/Pro-Am

Cecilia

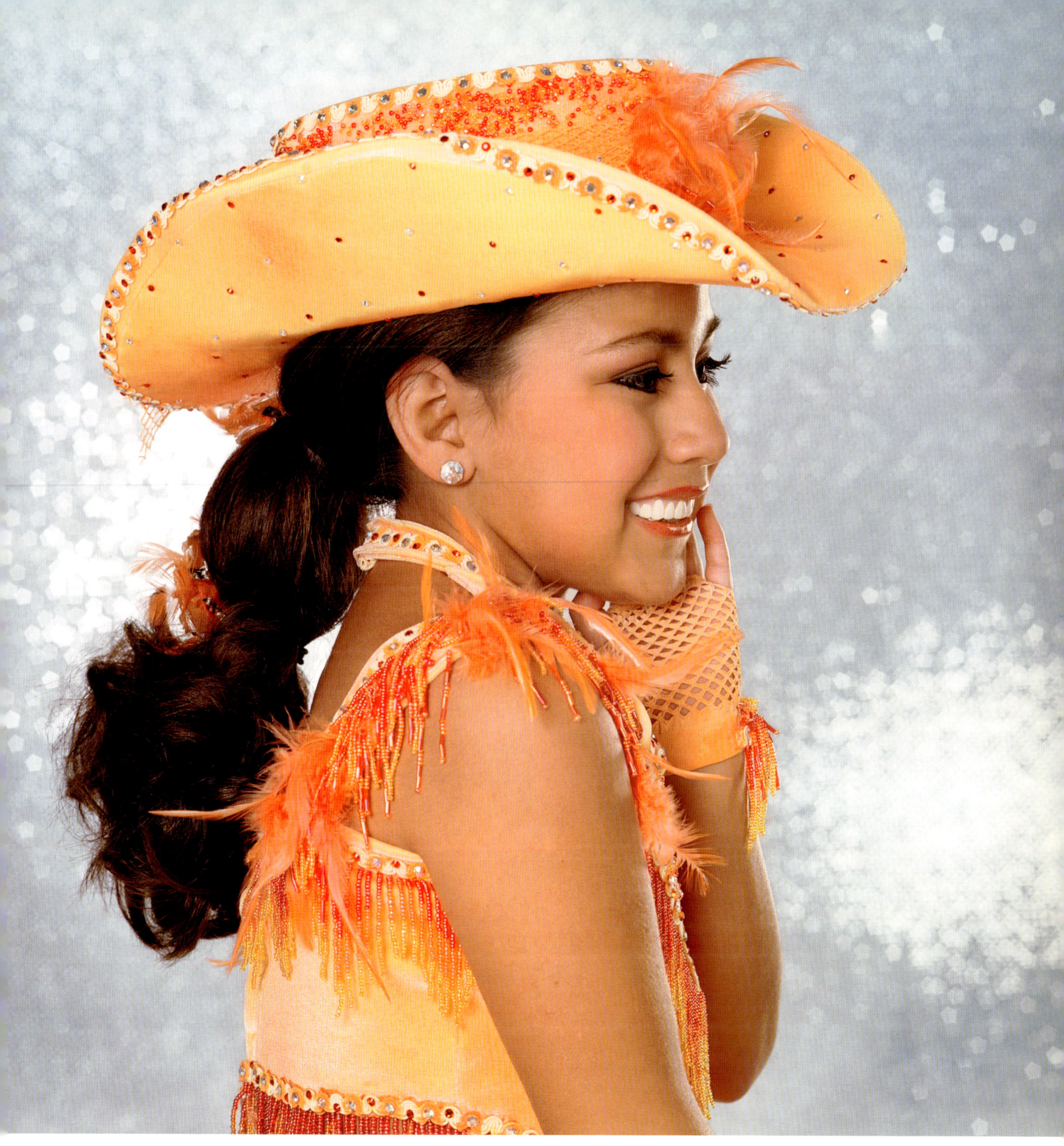

Age 7 × Santa Ana, California × 2005

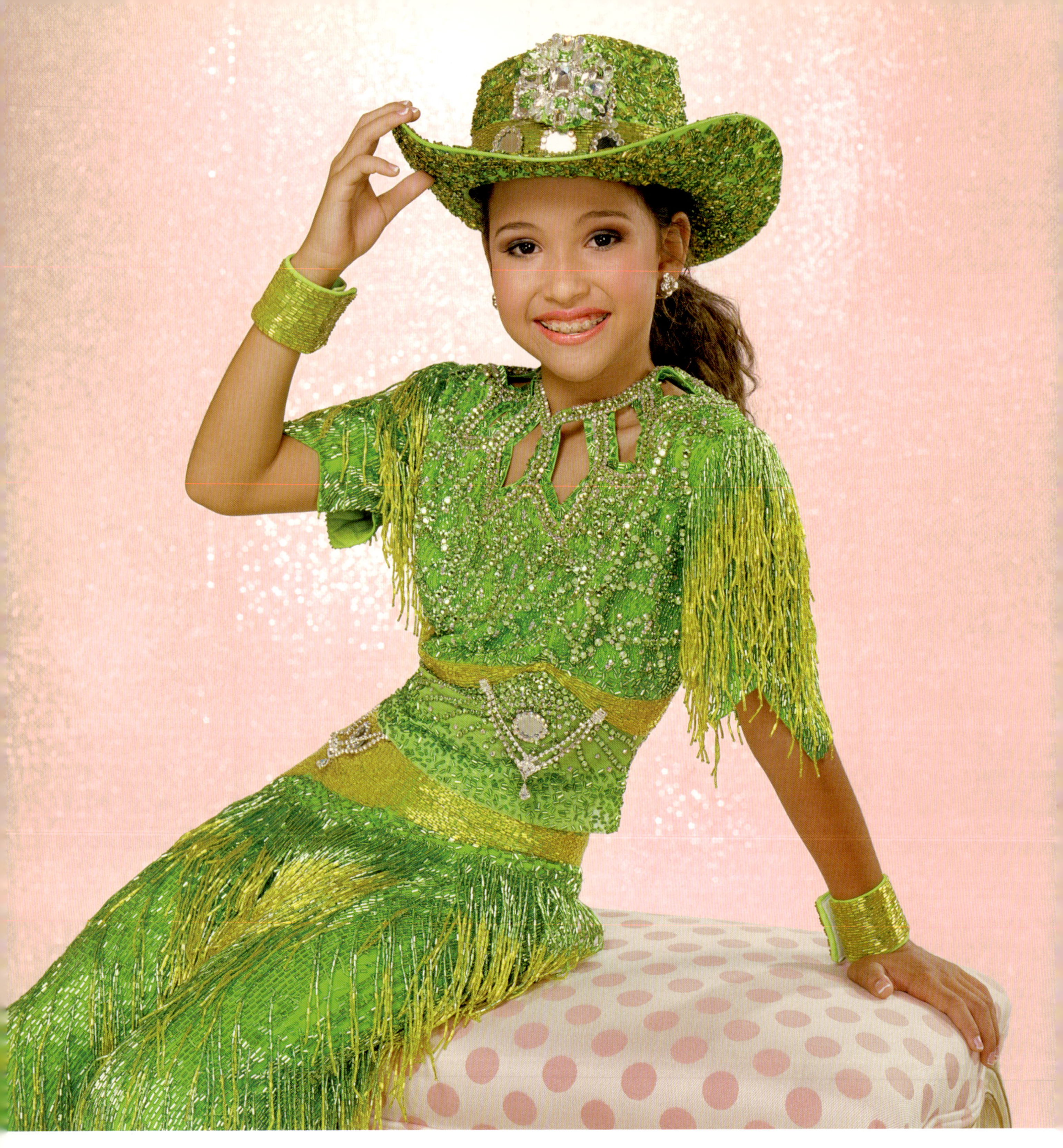

Heidi × Age 9 × Austin, Texas × 2005

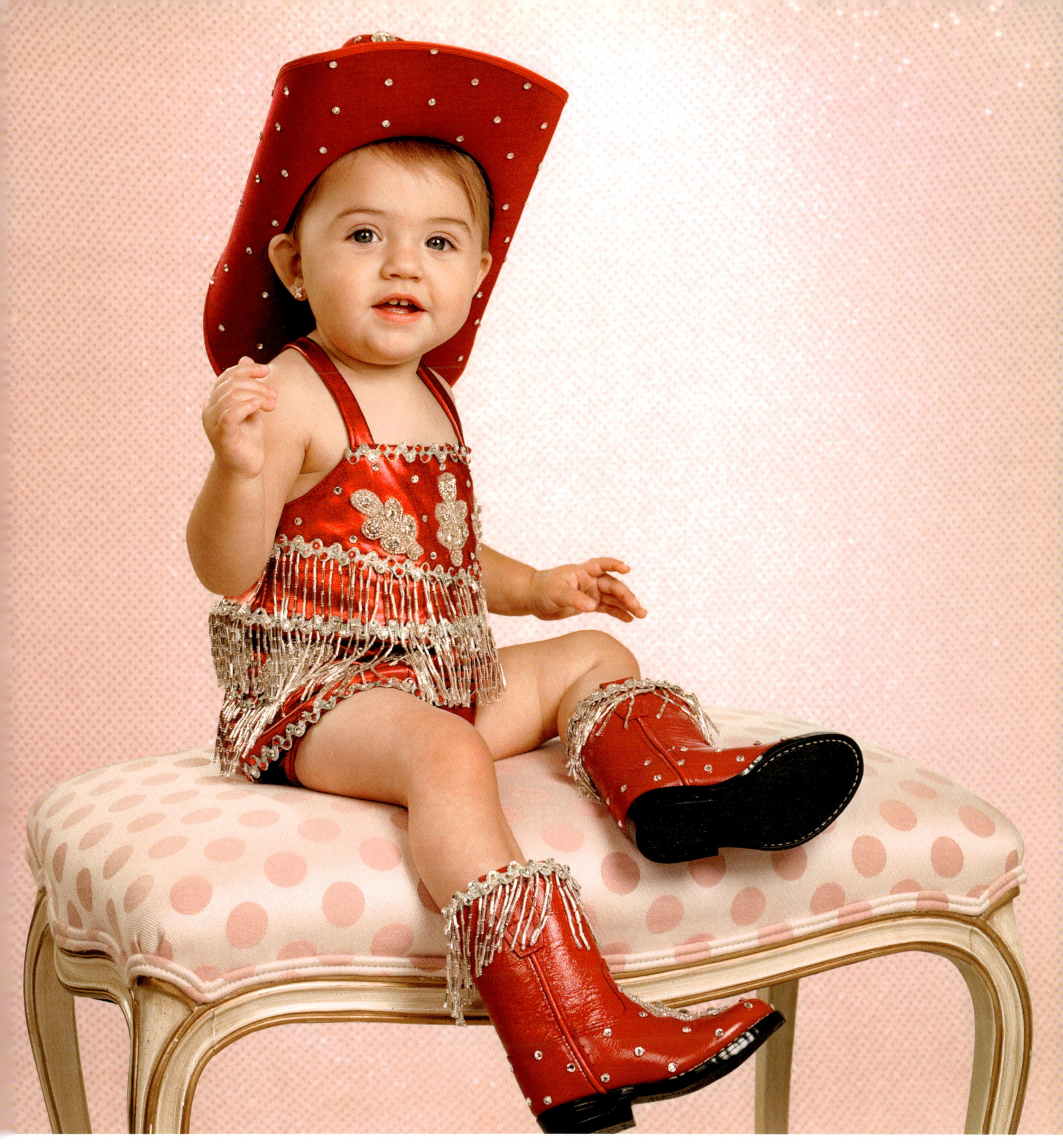

Gracie × Age 18 Months × Austin, Texas × 2005

Madison

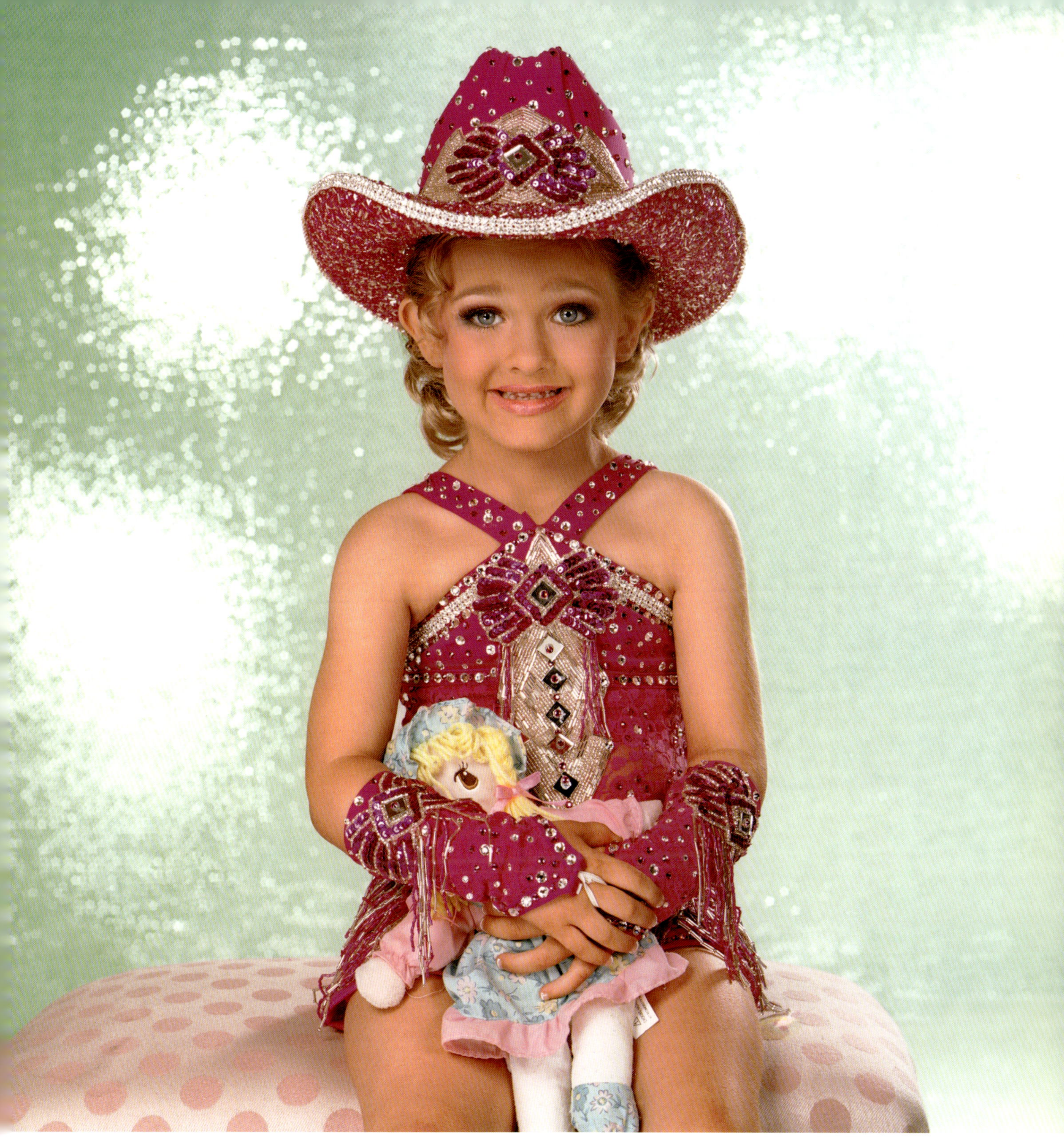

Age 4 ✕ Nashville, Tennessee ✕ 2008

Katarina

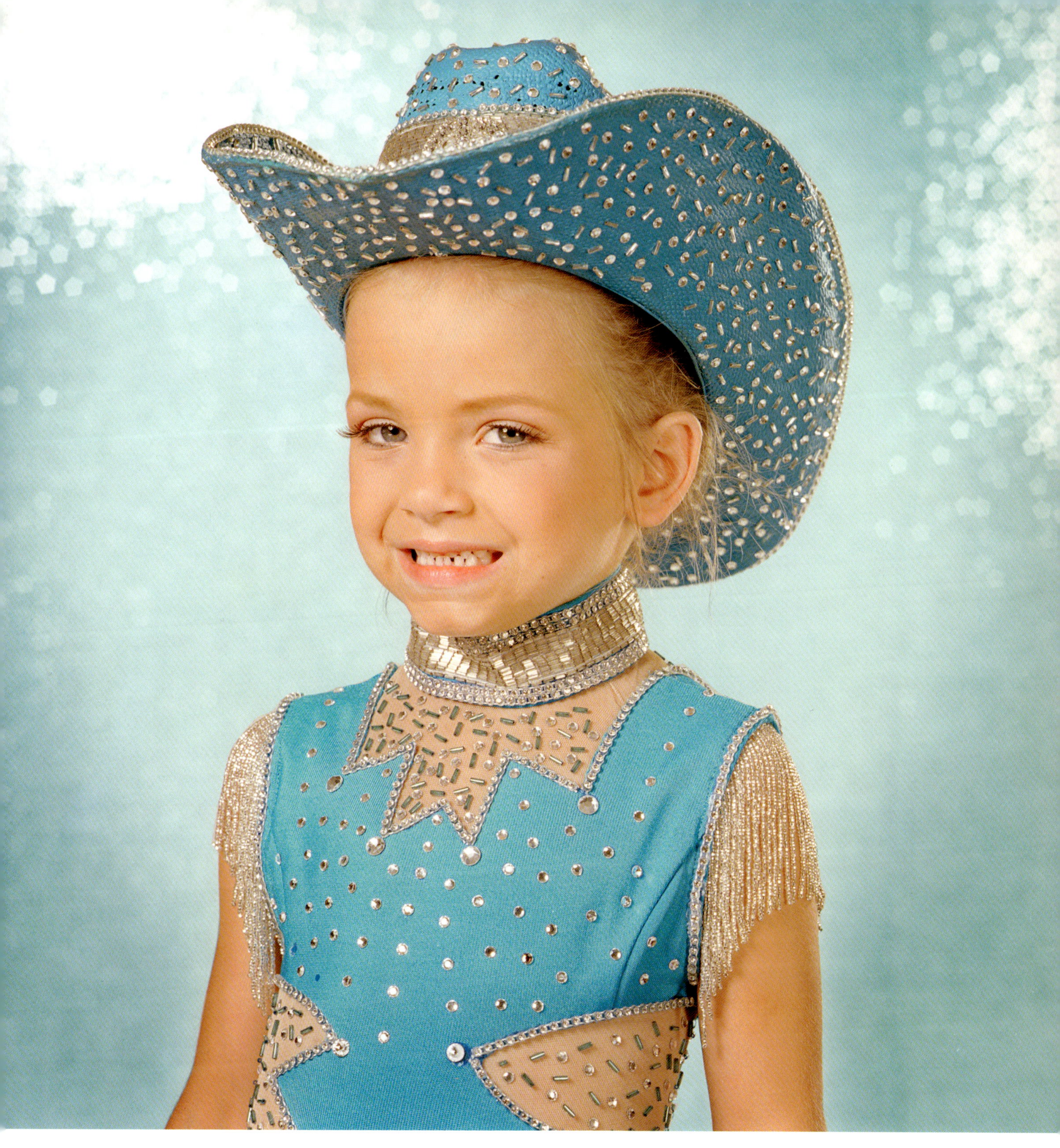

Age 5 × Las Vegas, Nevada × 2006

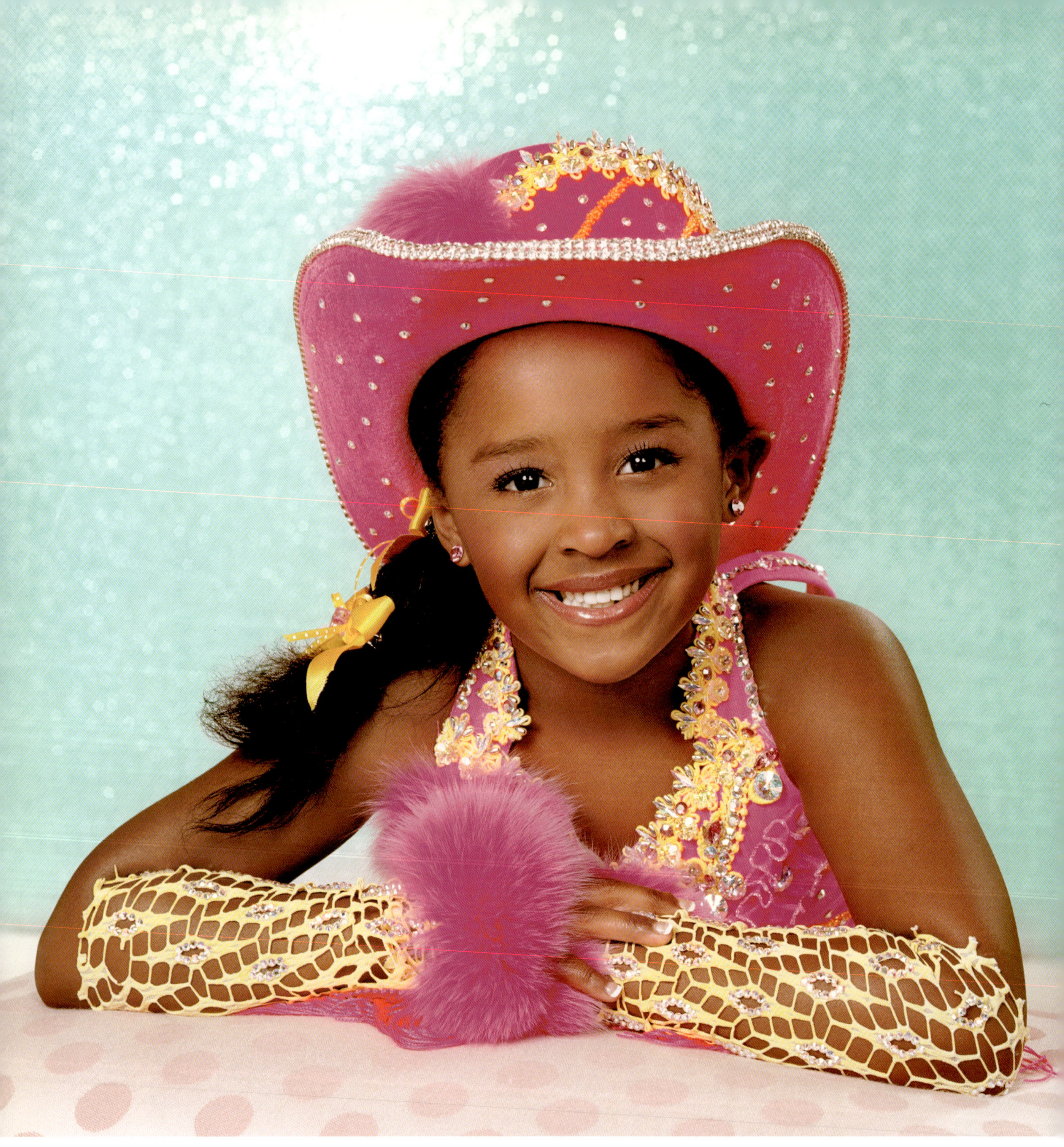

Kirrah

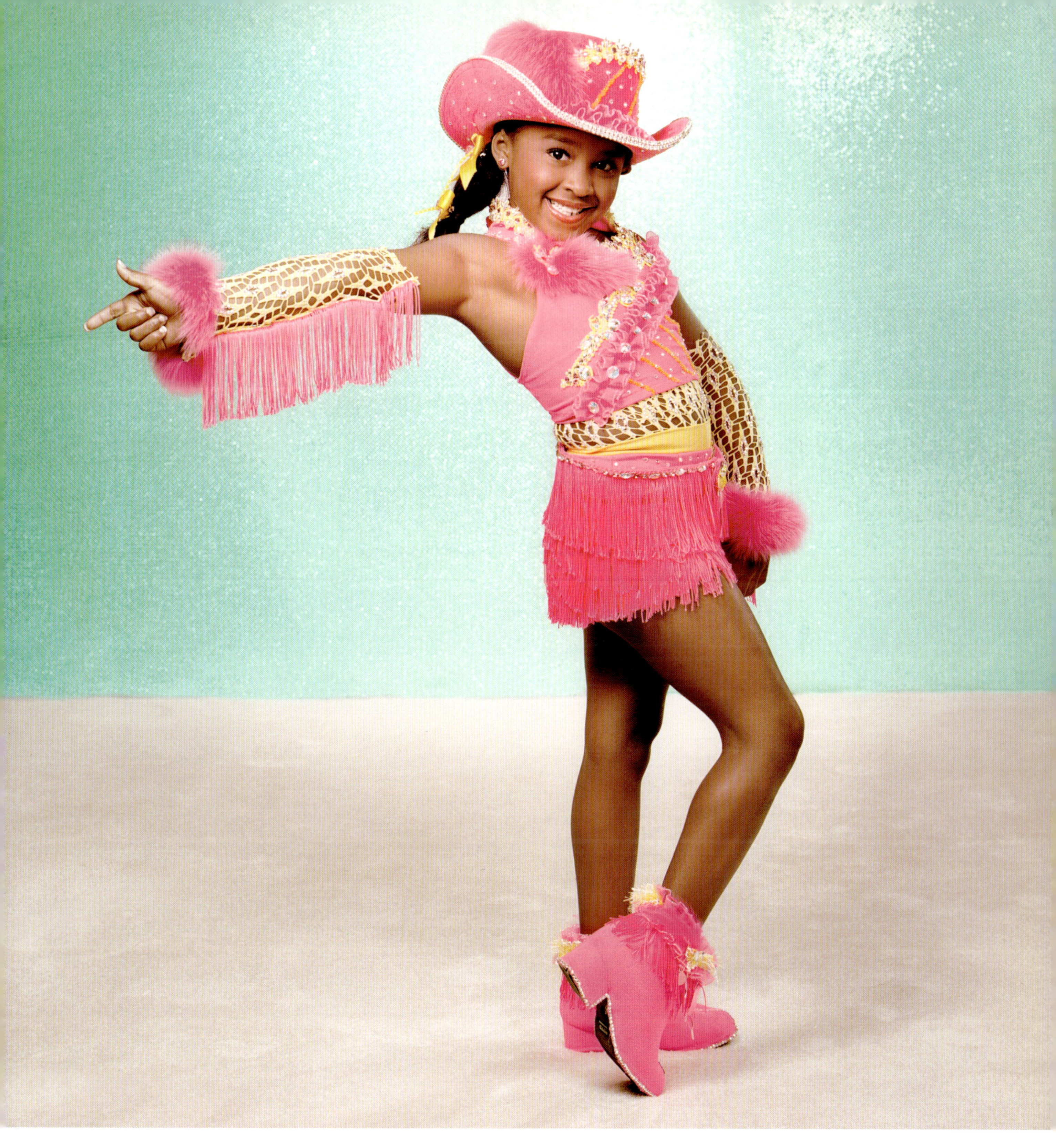

Age 5 · Austin, Texas · 2005

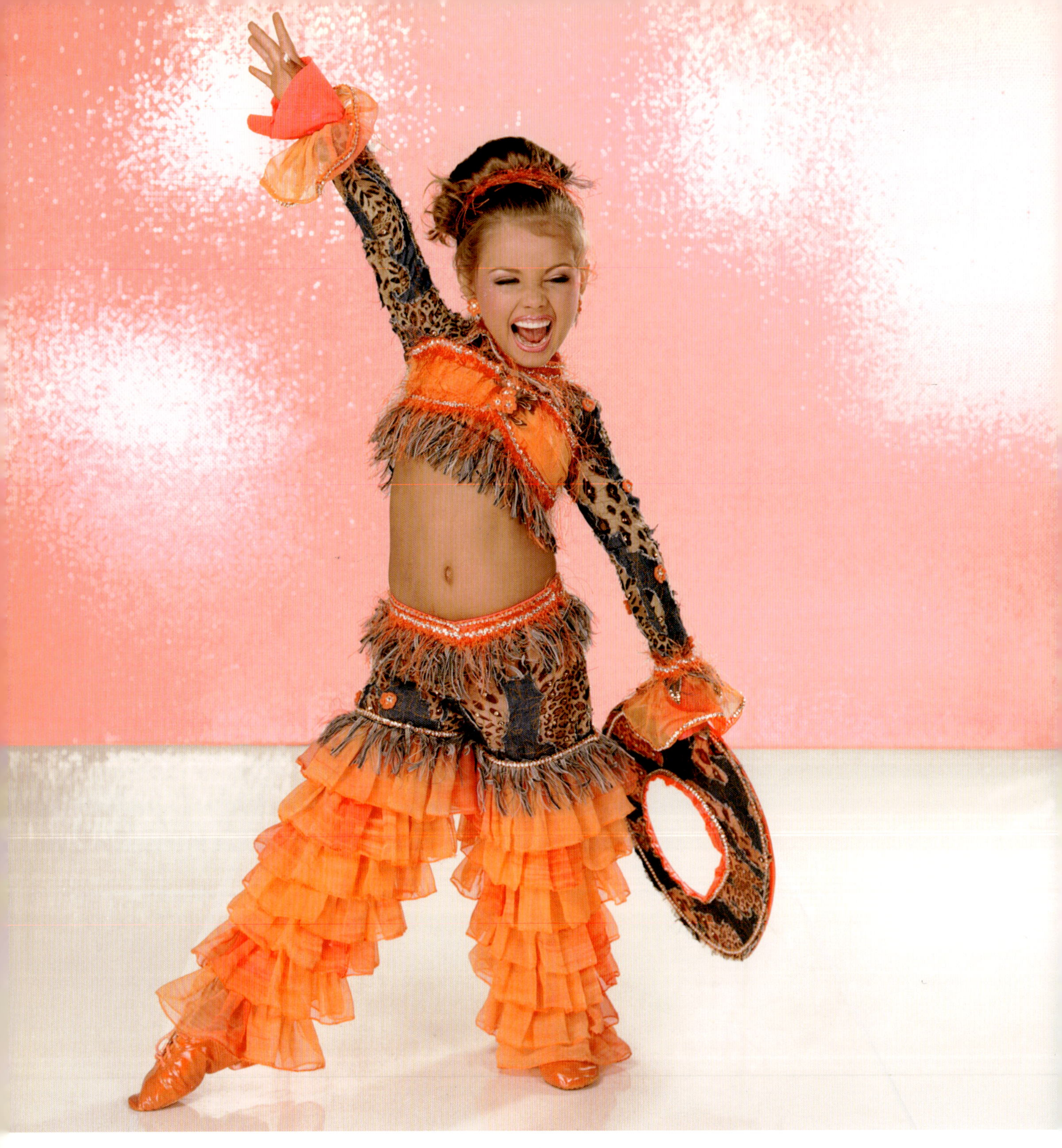

Tatum

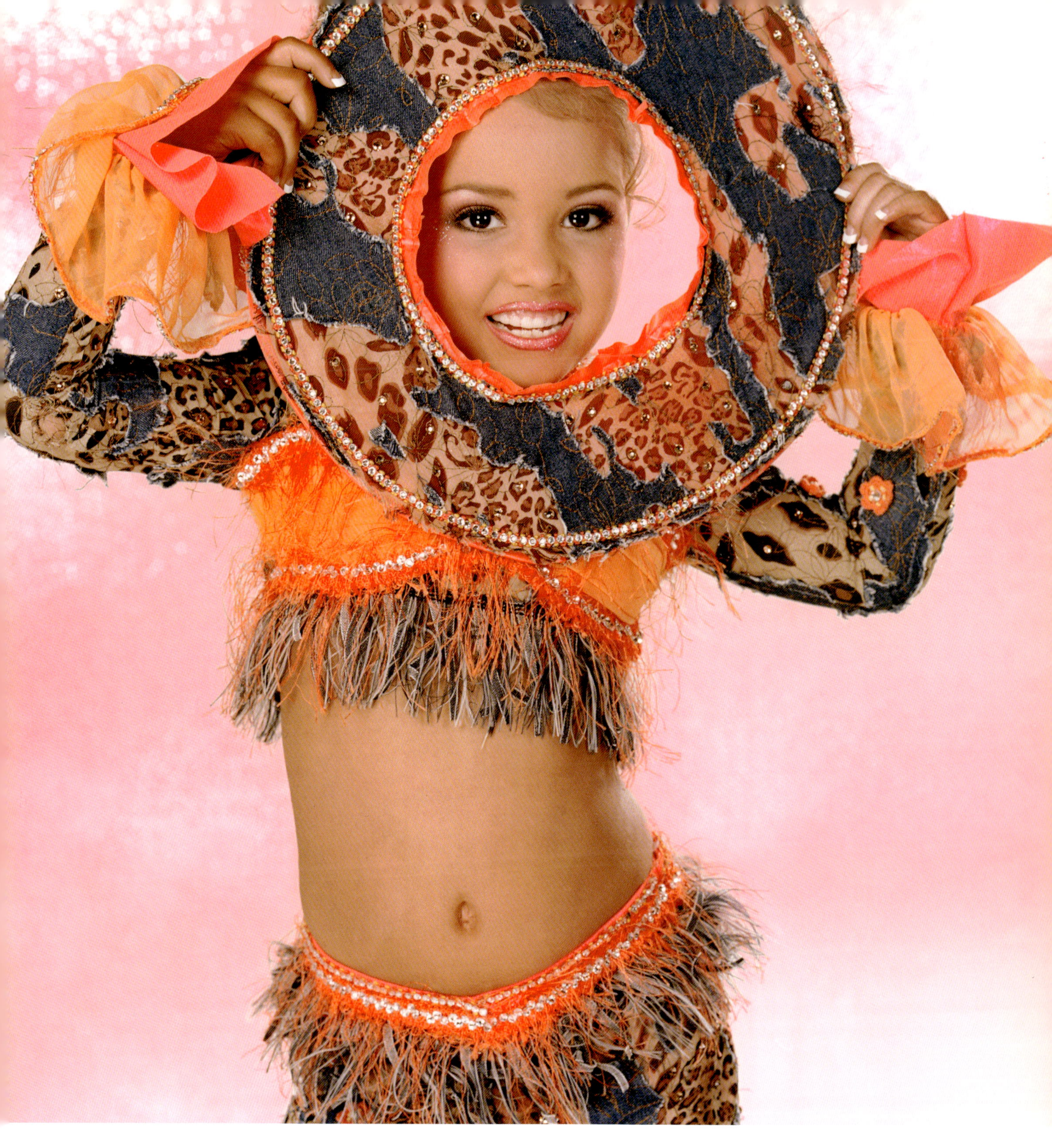

Age 5 × Nashville, Tennessee × 2008

Raylee

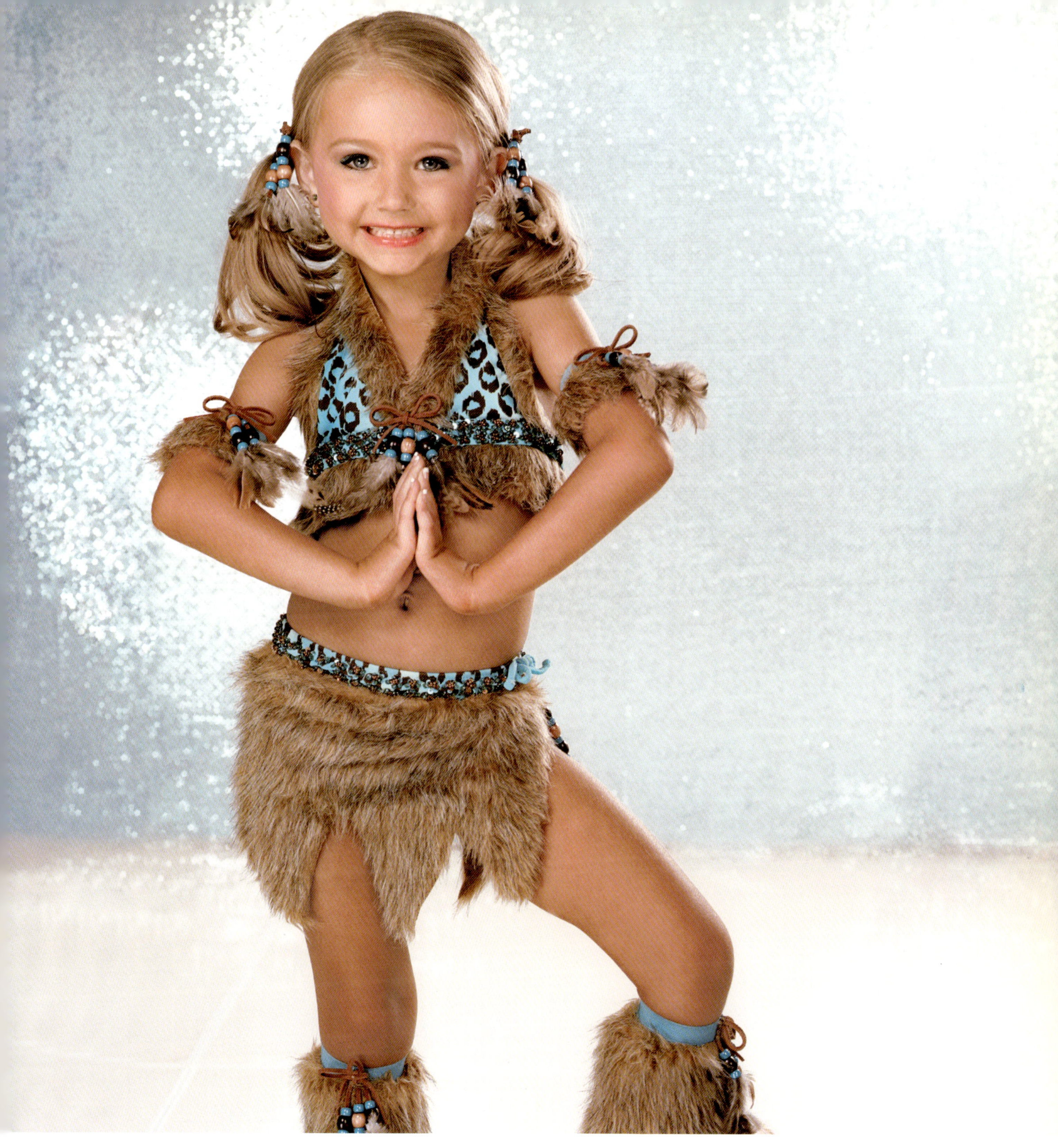

Age 5 ✶ Nashville, Tennessee ✶ 2008

Olivia

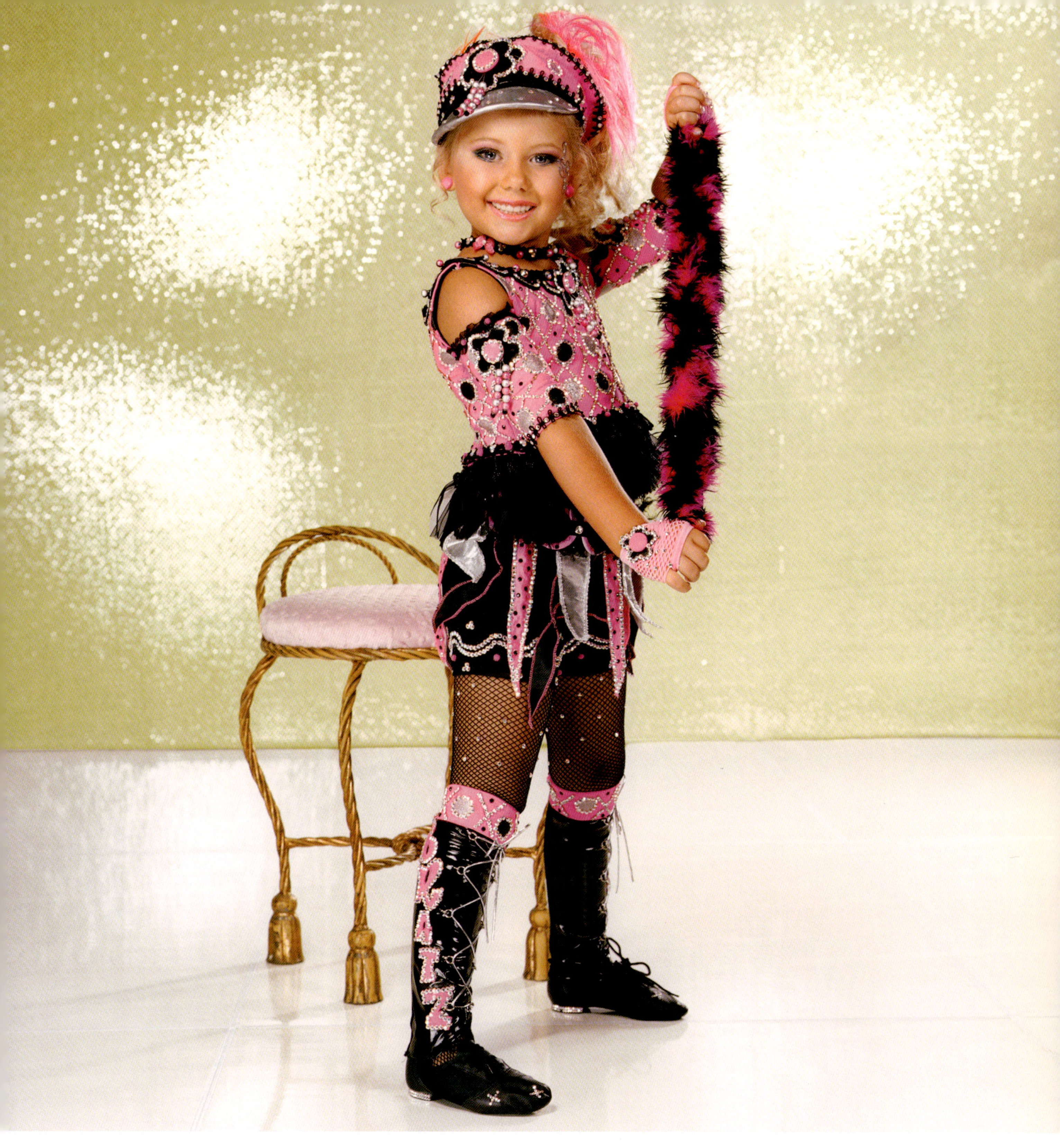

Age 5 × Nashville, Tennessee × 2008

Kaylie

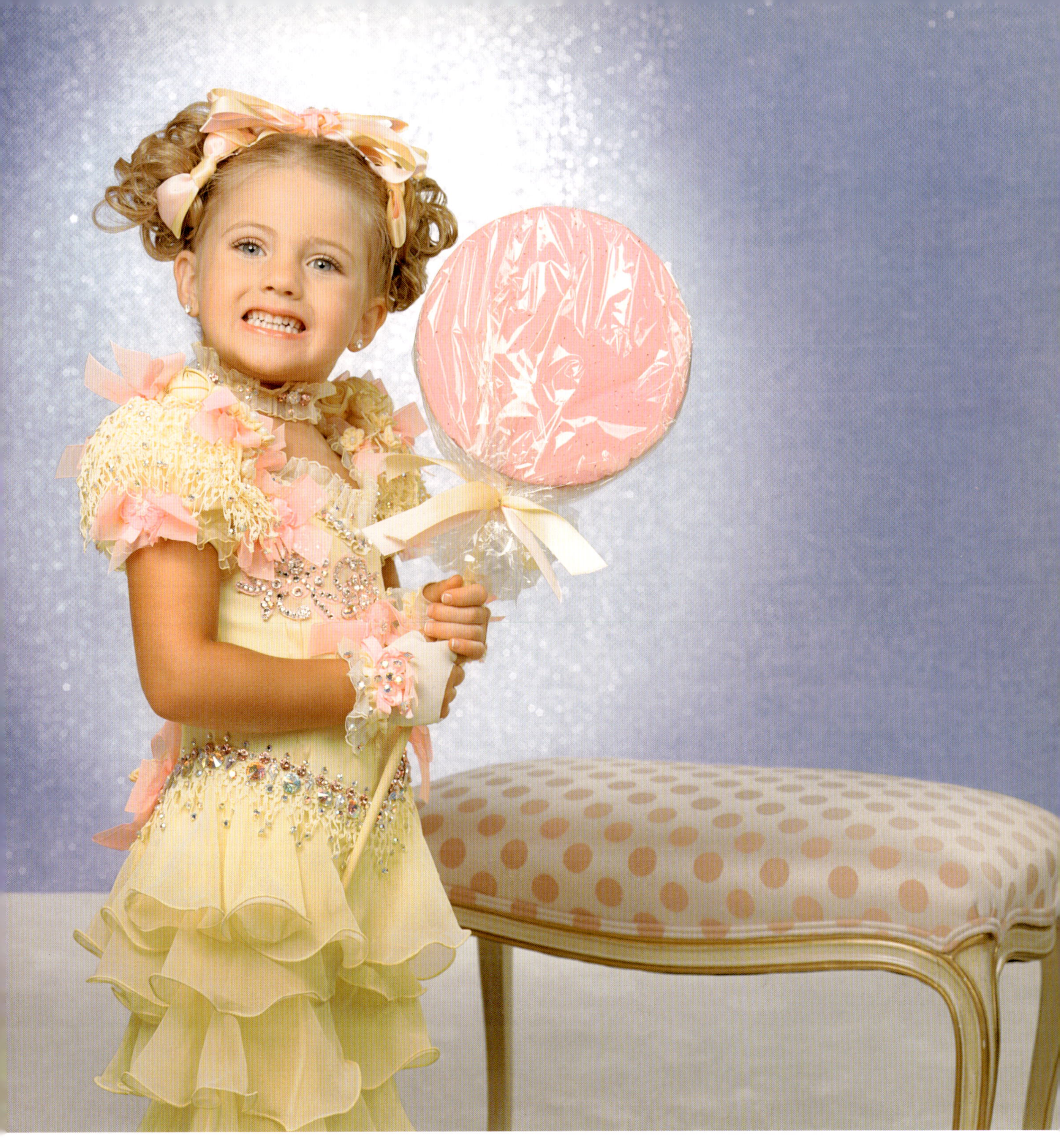

Age 3 × Austin, Texas × 2005

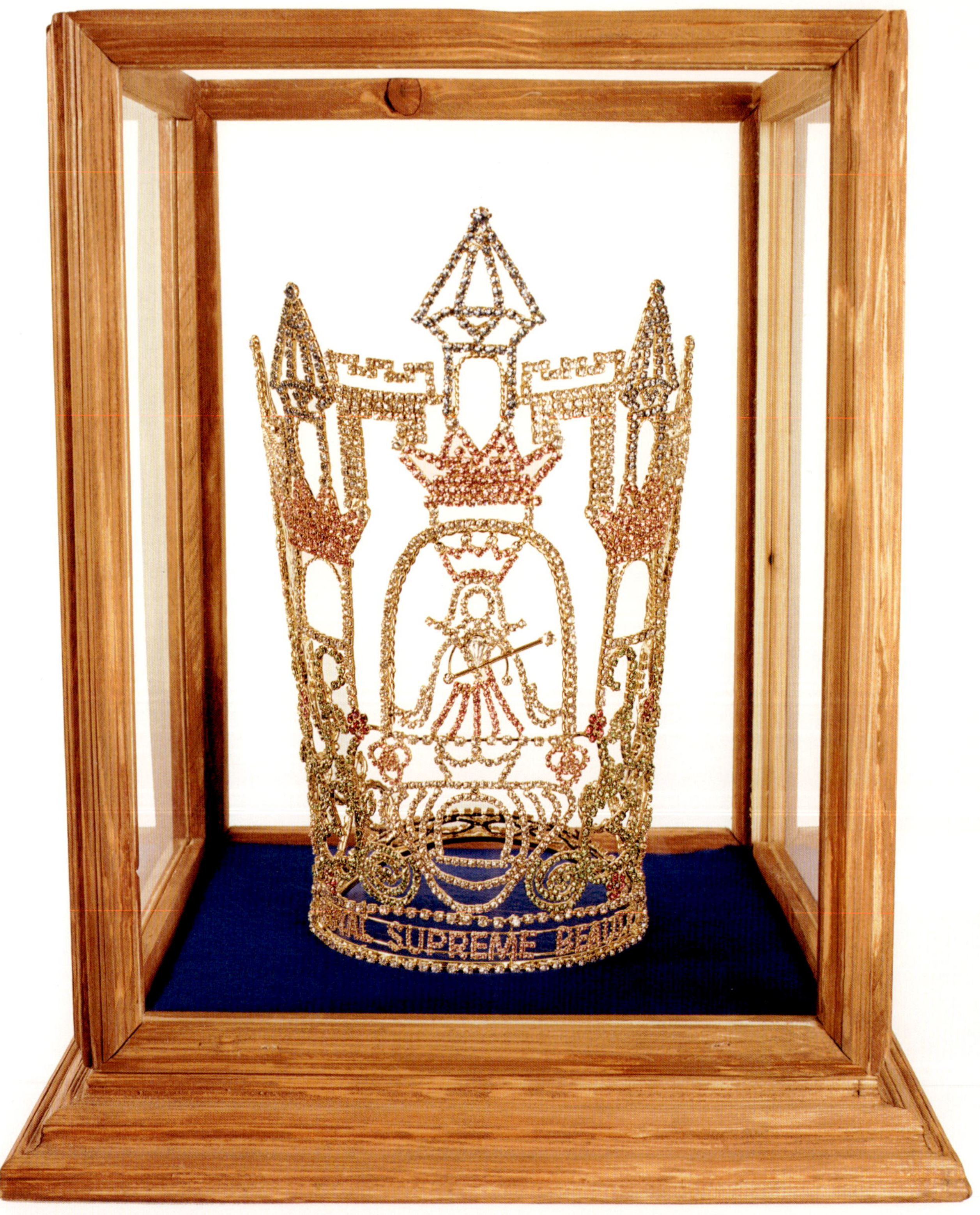
SUPREME

Hair & Makeup

Devan

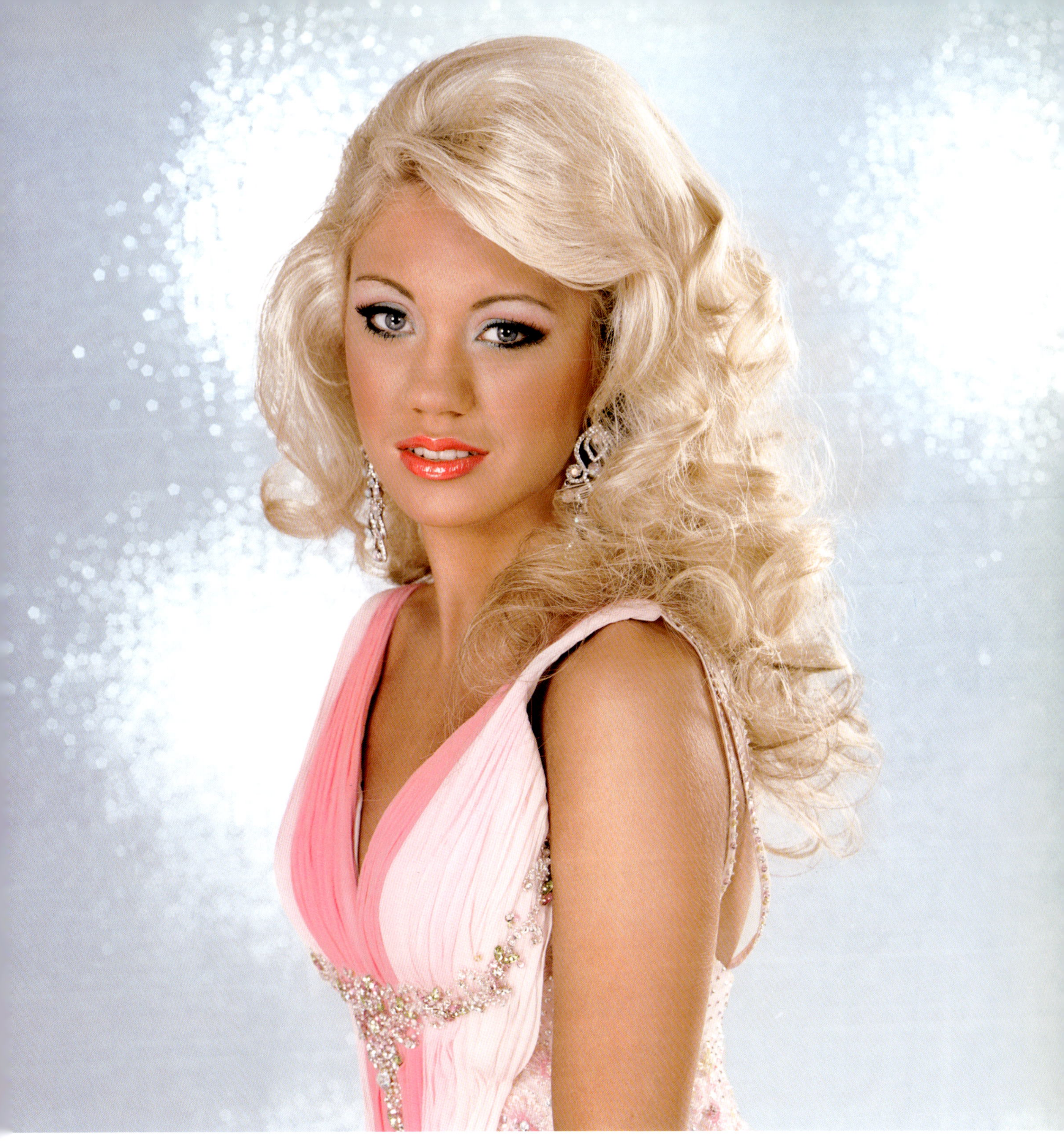

Age 13 × Nashville, Tennessee × 2008

Krysten

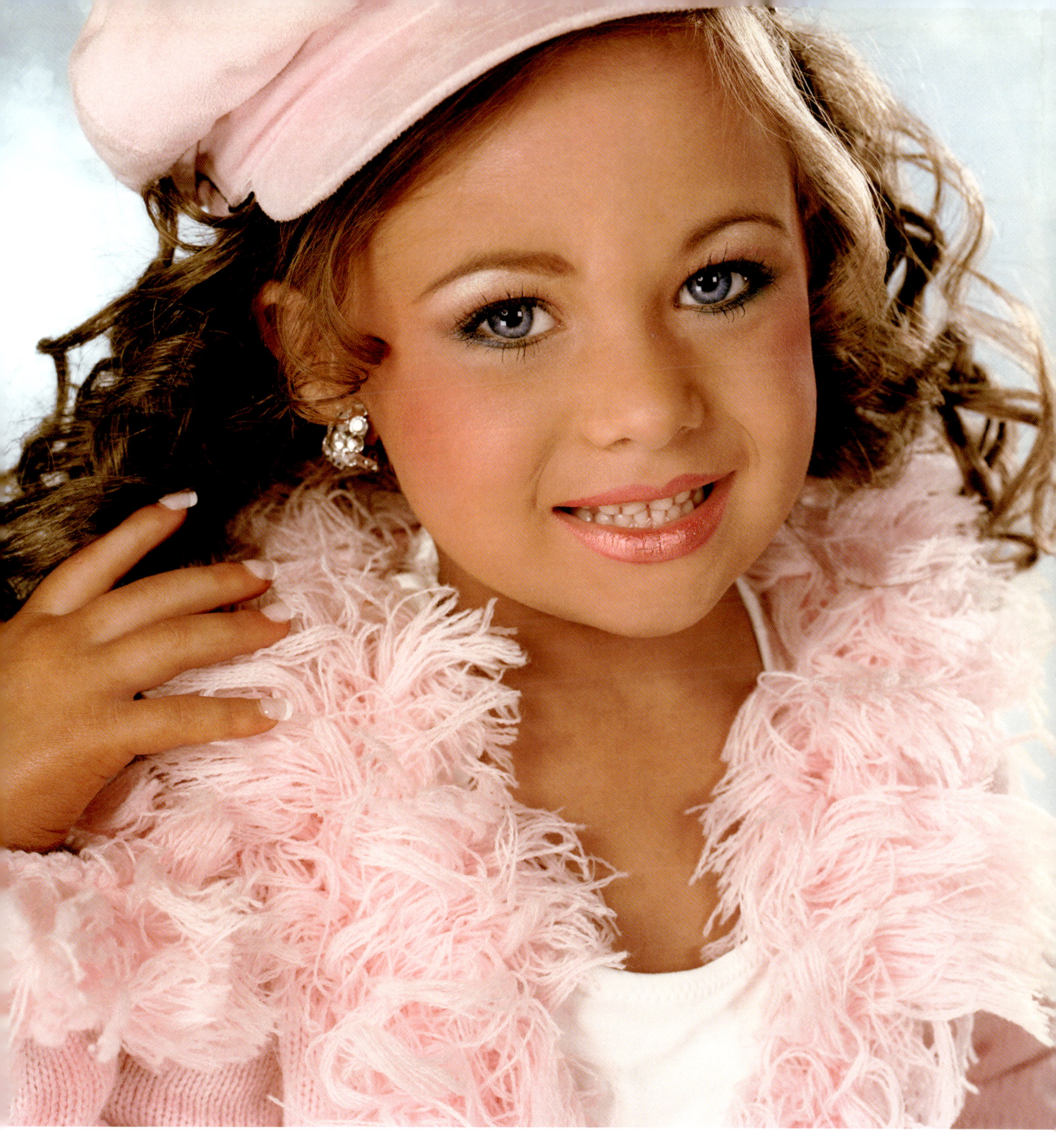

Age 5 × Nashville, Tennessee × 2008

Kendra

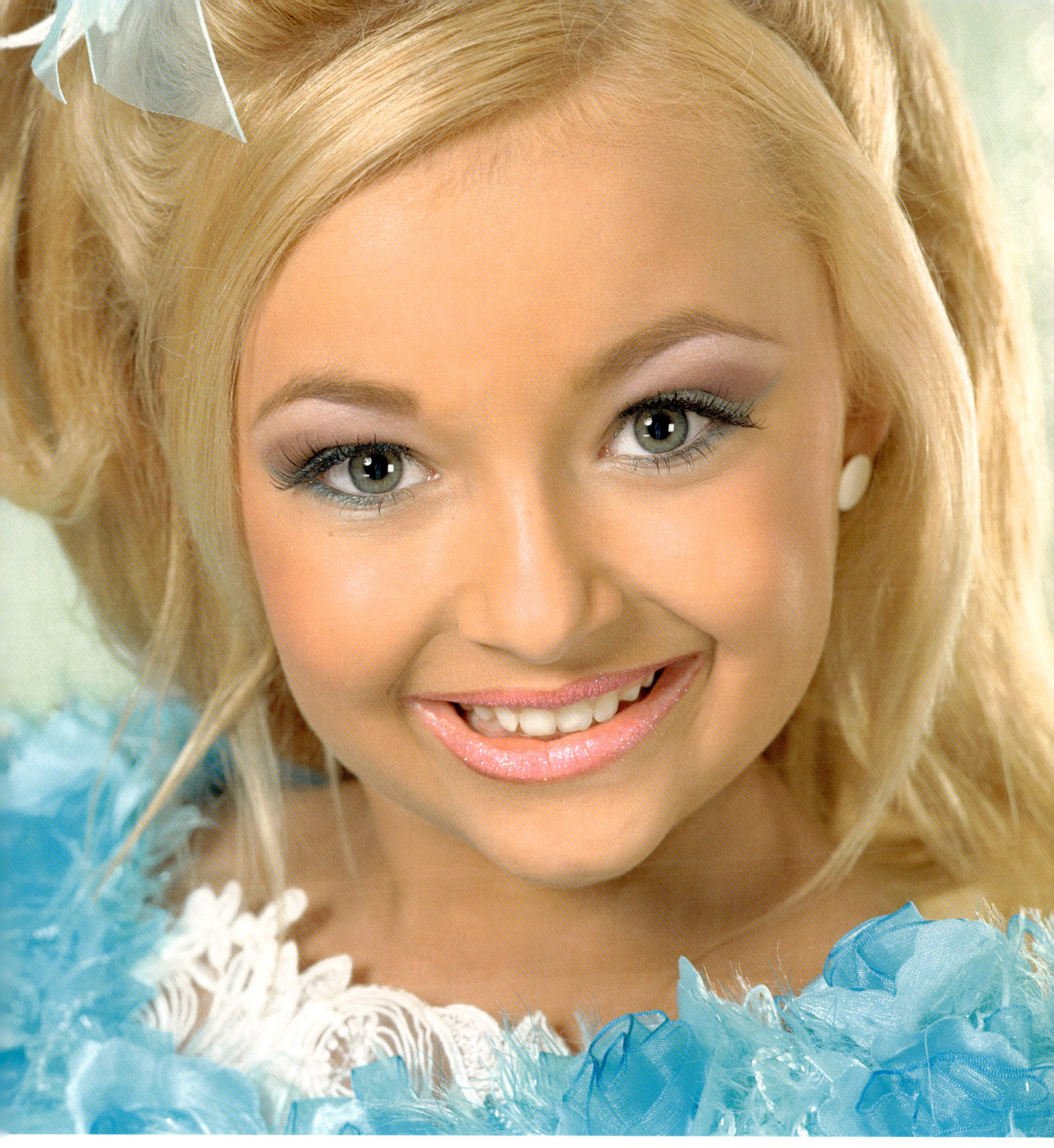

Age 10 × Las Vegas, Nevada × 2006

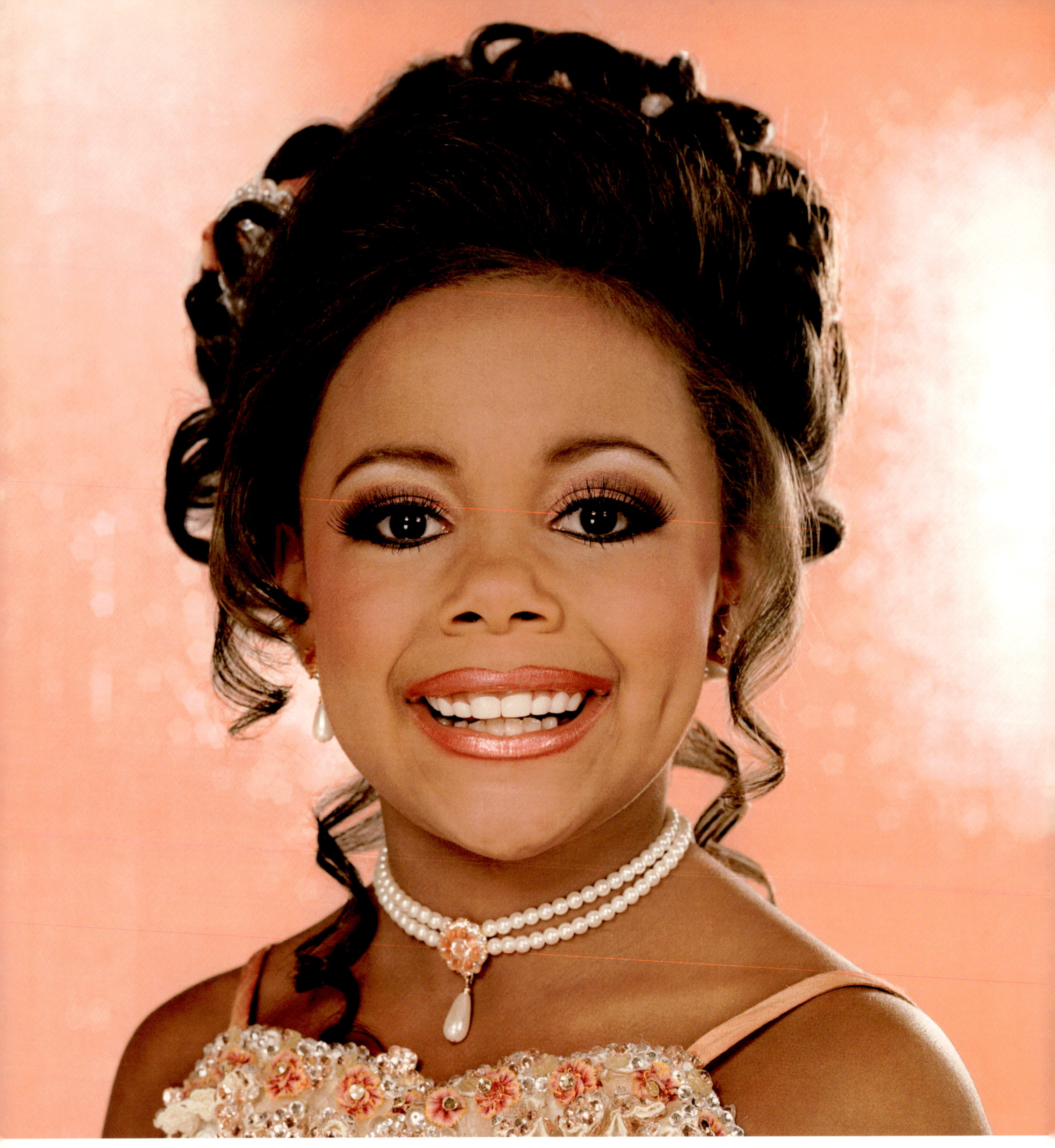

Sydney

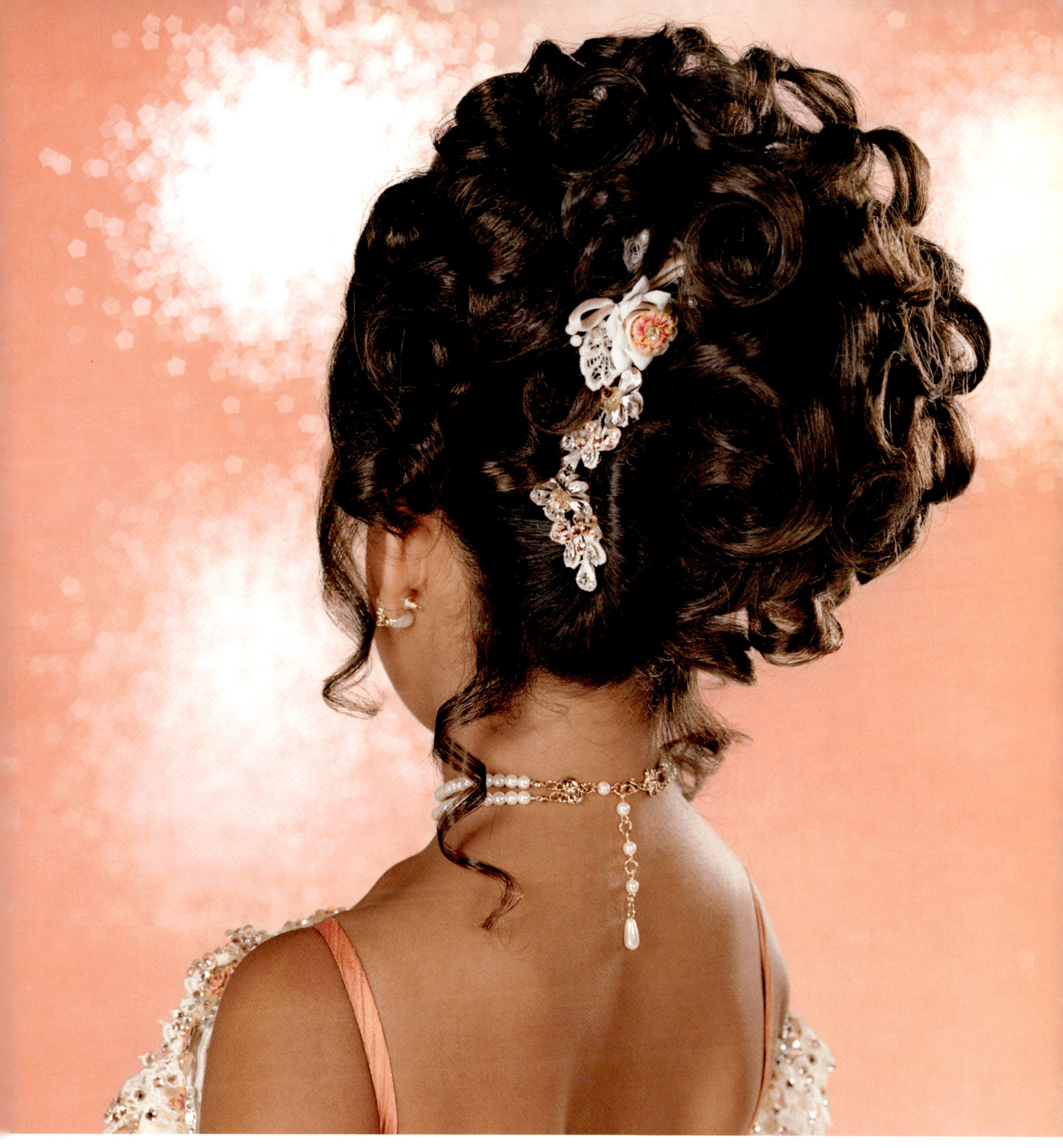

Age 8 ✶ Nashville, Tennessee ✶ 2008

Marilyn

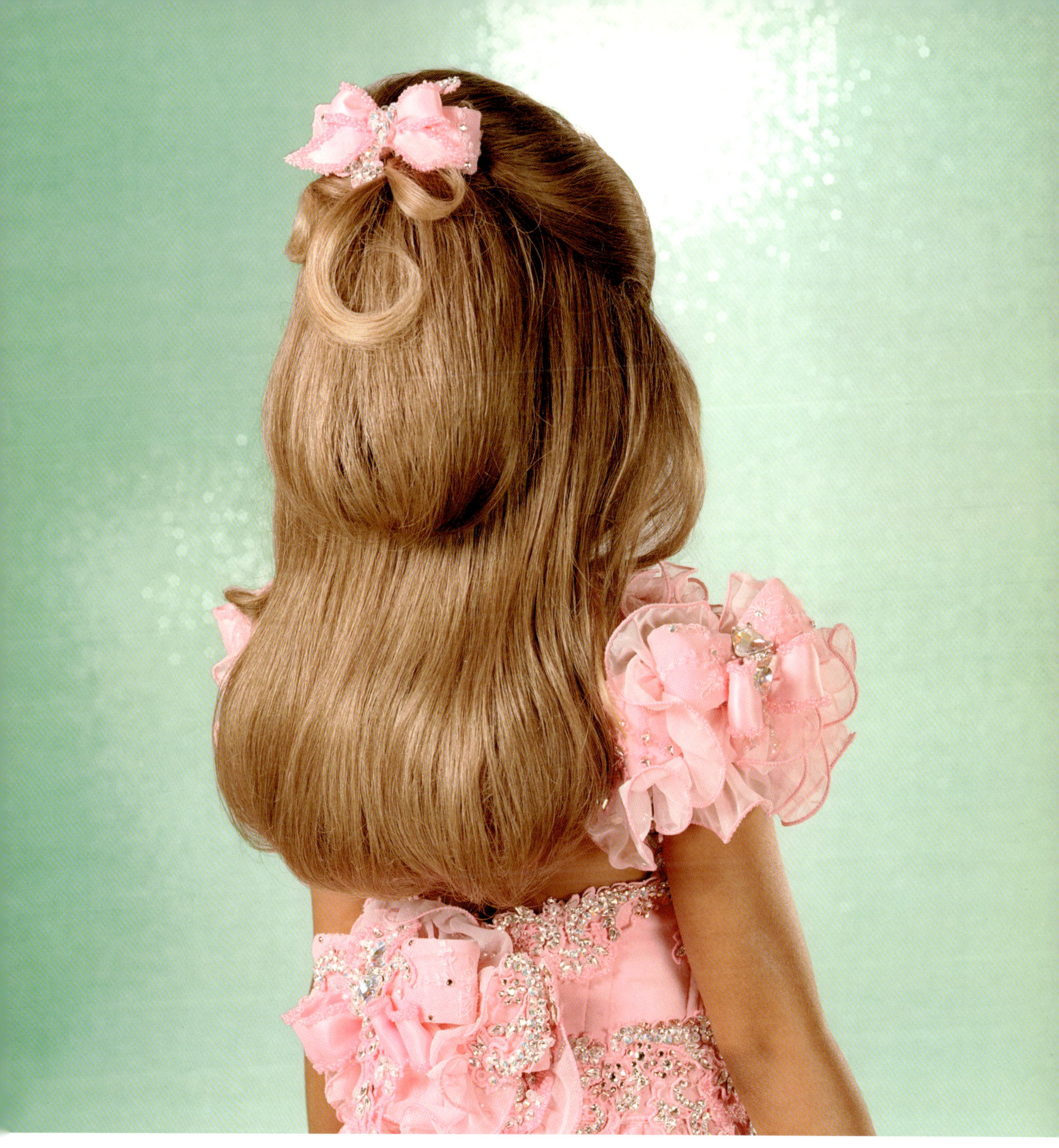

Age 8 × Las Vegas, Nevada × 2006

Allison

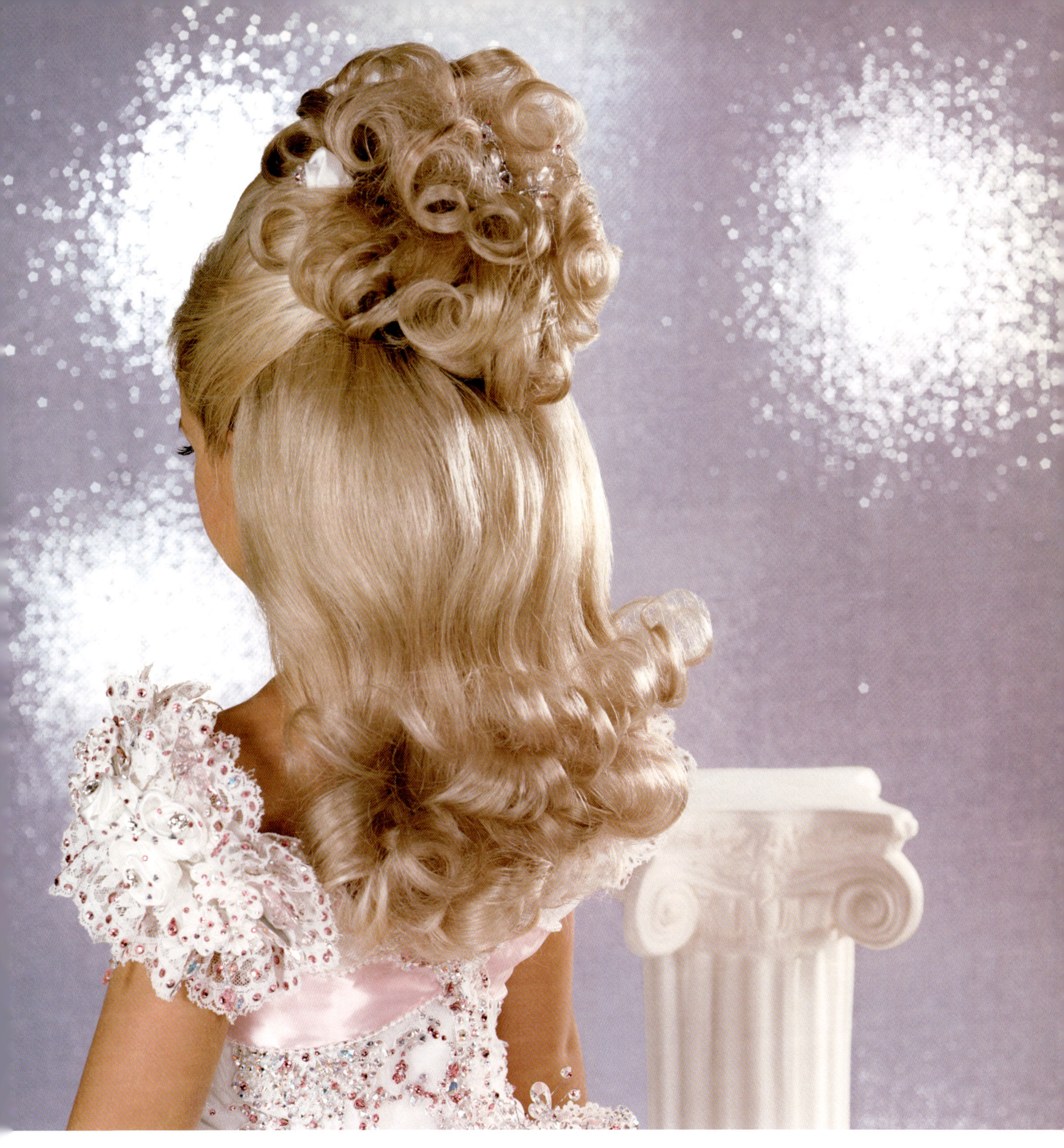

Age 10 × Nashville, Tennessee × 2008

Annabelle

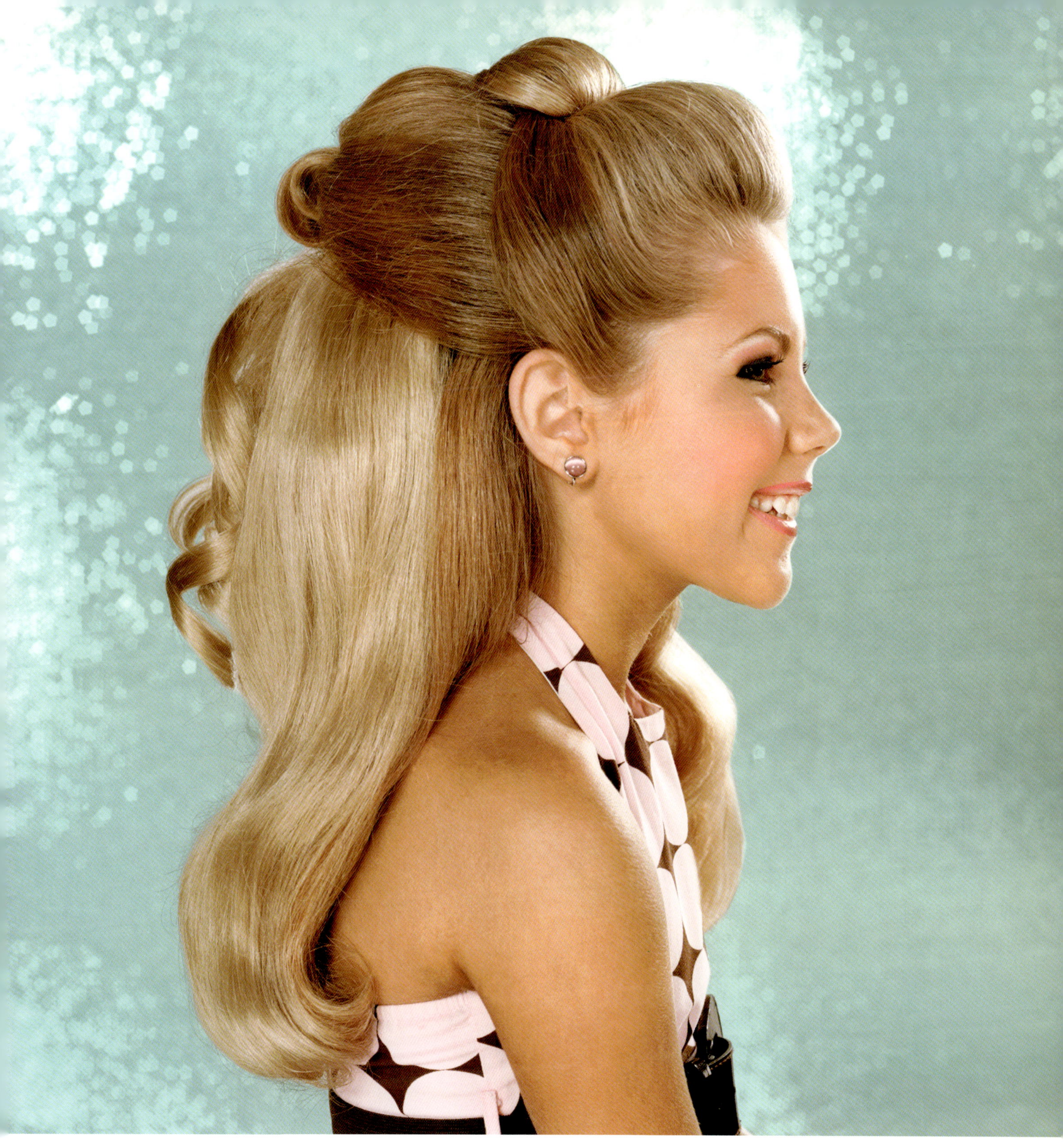

Age 10 × Nashville, Tennessee × 2008

Annabelle

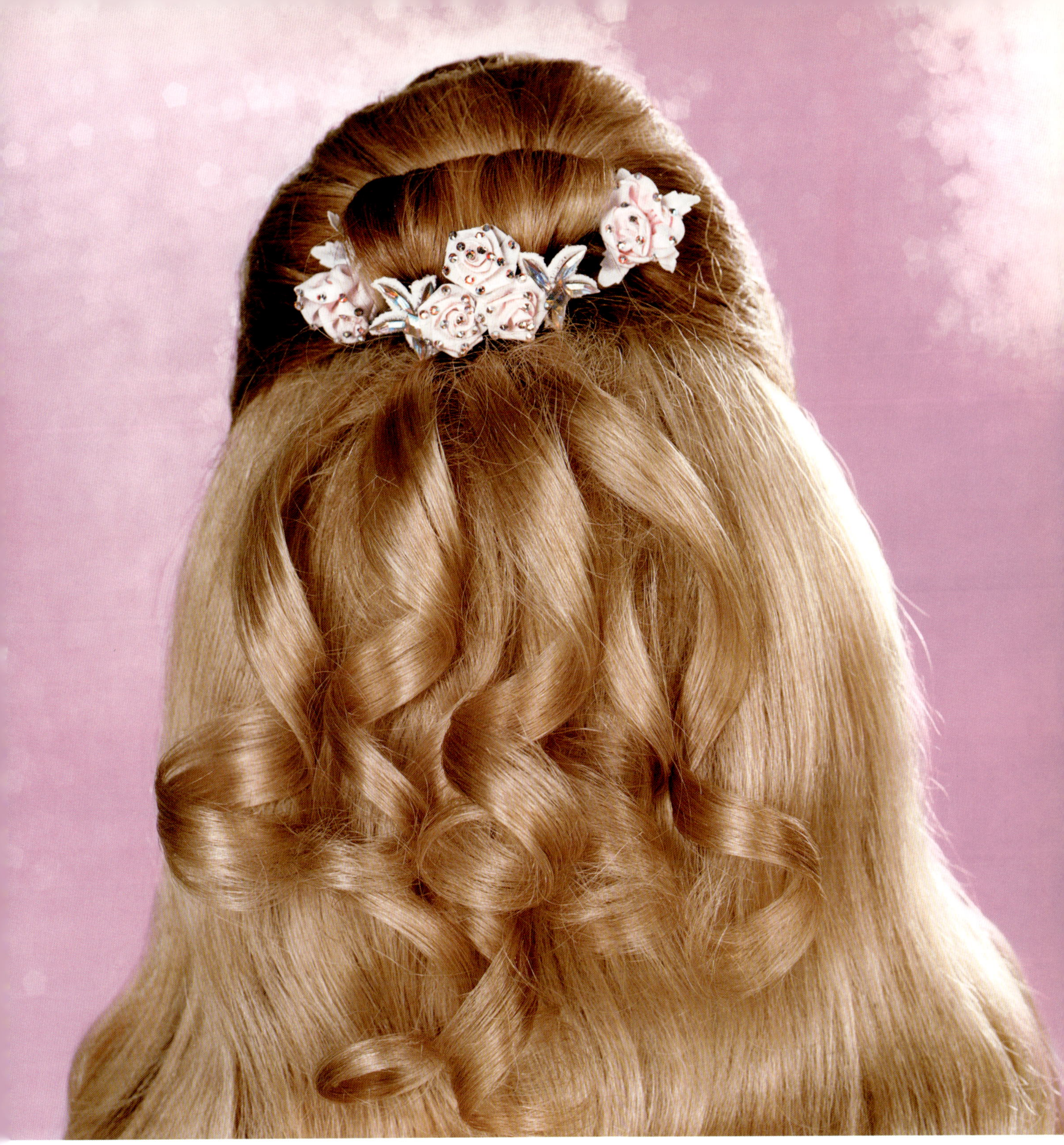

Age 10 ⋆ Nashville, Tennessee ⋆ 2008

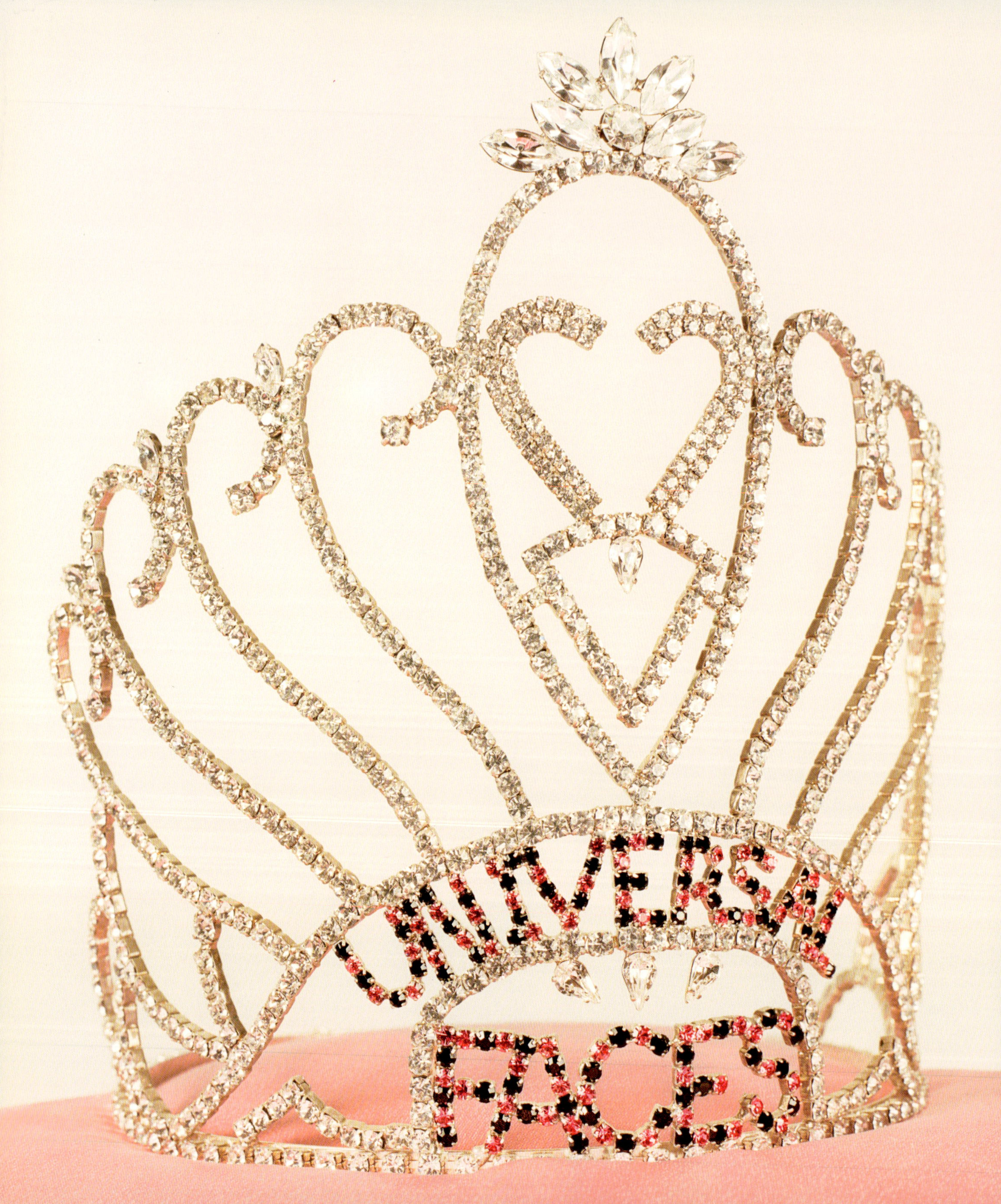
UNIVERSAL
FACES

Crowning

Universal Miss Glamour Queen
Universal Miss Beauty Supreme
National Beauty Queen
National Dream Doll Queen
National Queen
National Overall Most Beautiful
National Overall Pro-Am
Overall Beauty Supreme
Overall Model Supreme
Grand Model Supreme
Super Model Supreme
Ultimate Supreme
Swimwear Supreme
Talent Supreme
Grand Talent Supreme
Grand Supreme
Baby Grand
Mega Grand Supreme
Novice Mega Grand Supreme

Majestic Grand Supreme
Imperial Grand Supreme
Mini Grand Supreme
Grand Supreme Beauty
Royal Supreme Beauty
Beauty Supreme
Beauty Queen
Supreme Dream Doll Queen
Queen of Queens
Lifetime Queen of Queens
Universal Queen of Queens
Glitz Photo Supreme
Beauty Photogenic Supreme
Cover Miss Supreme
Front Cover/Centerfold
Overall Photogenic
Overall Sweetest Face
All American Angel
All American Miss

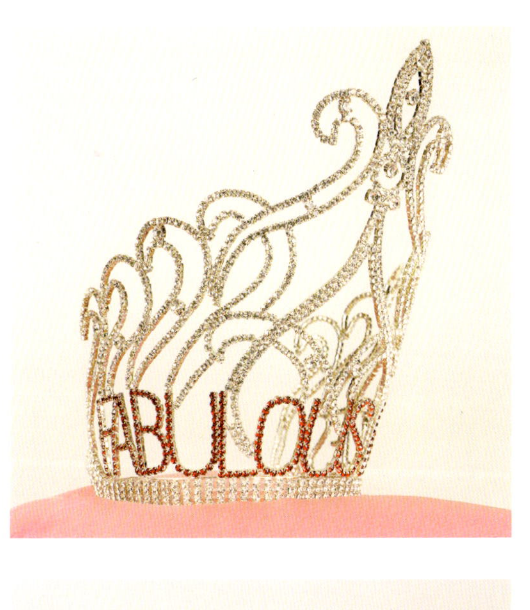

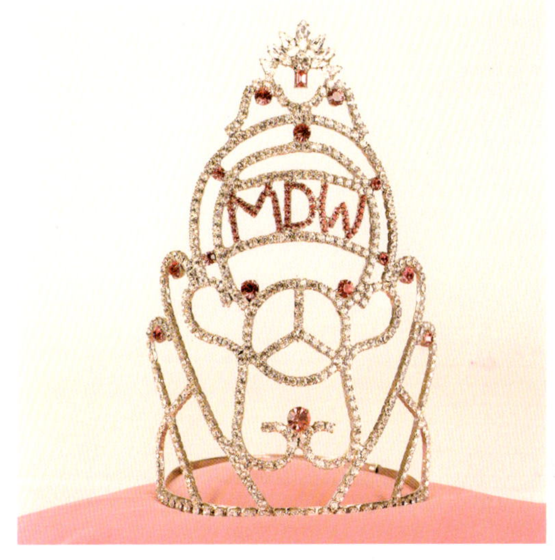
MDW

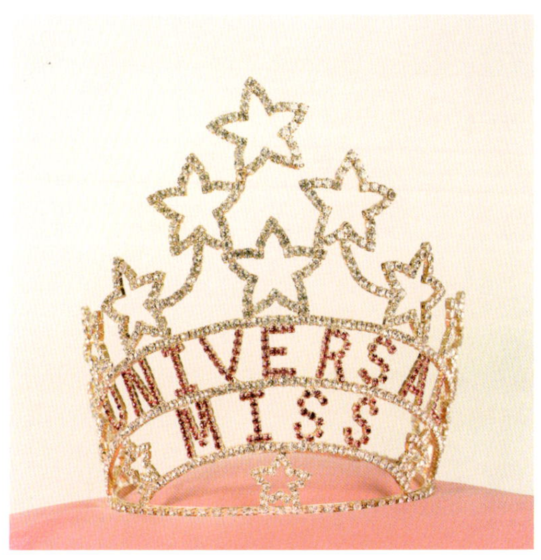
MISS

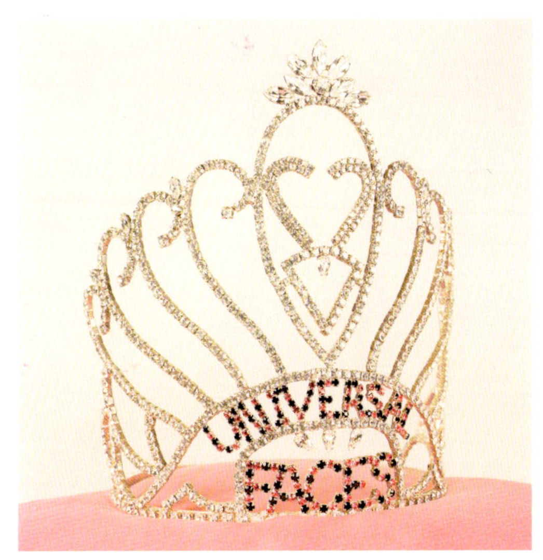
FACES

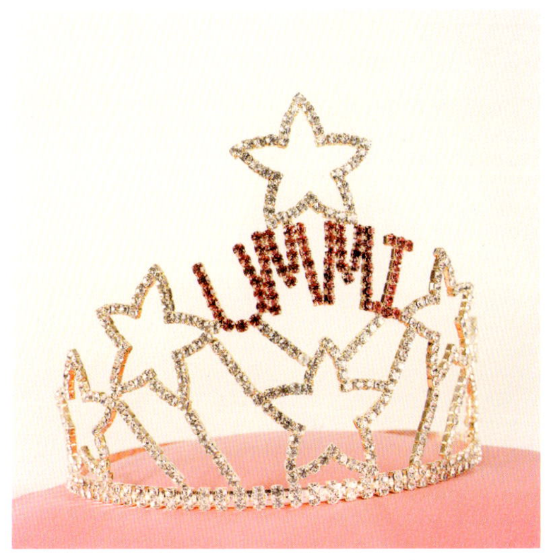

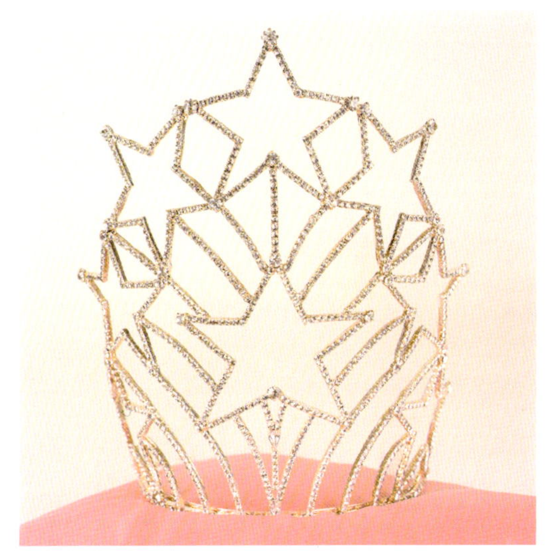

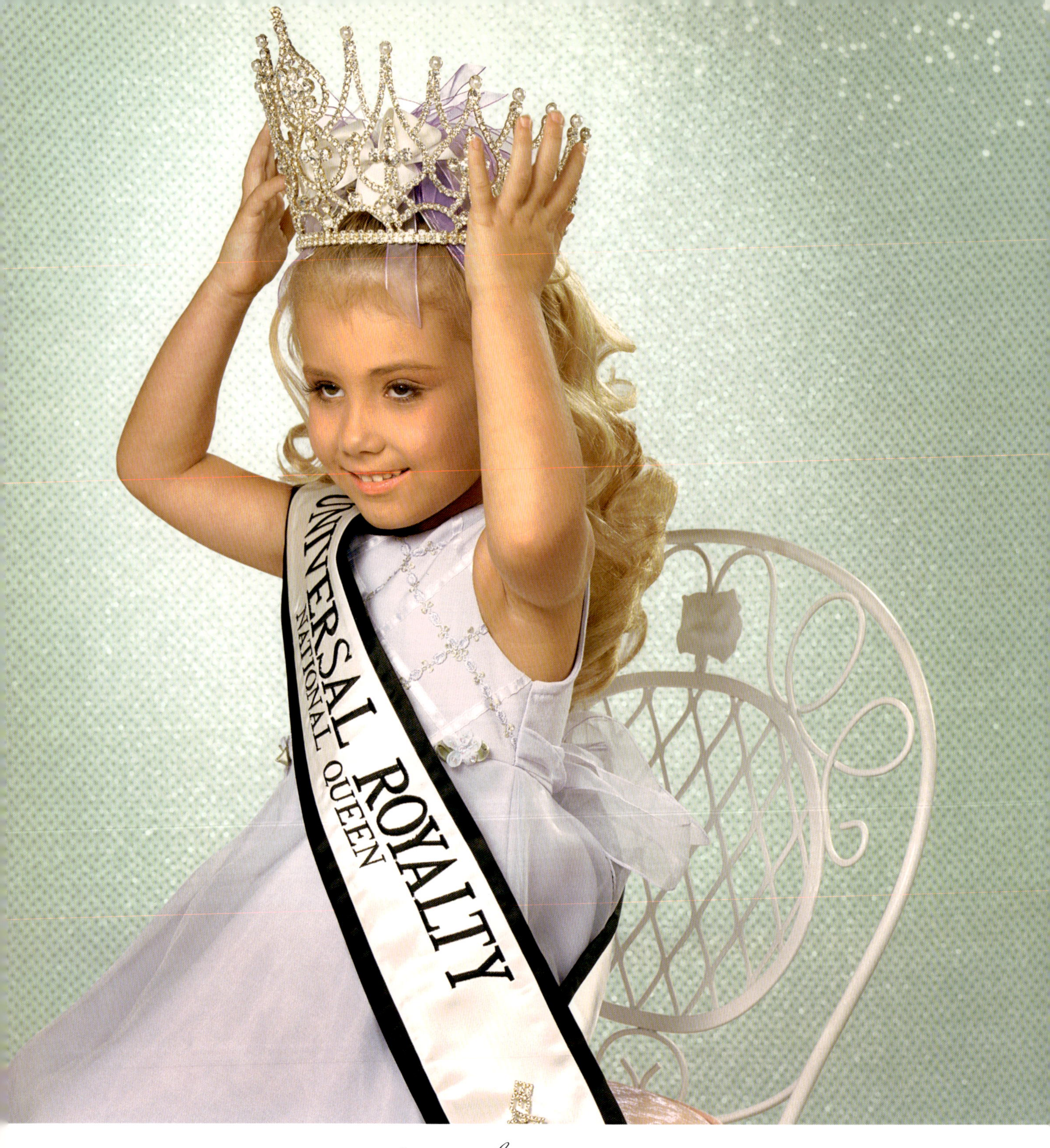

Savannah × Age 4 × Austin, Texas × 2005

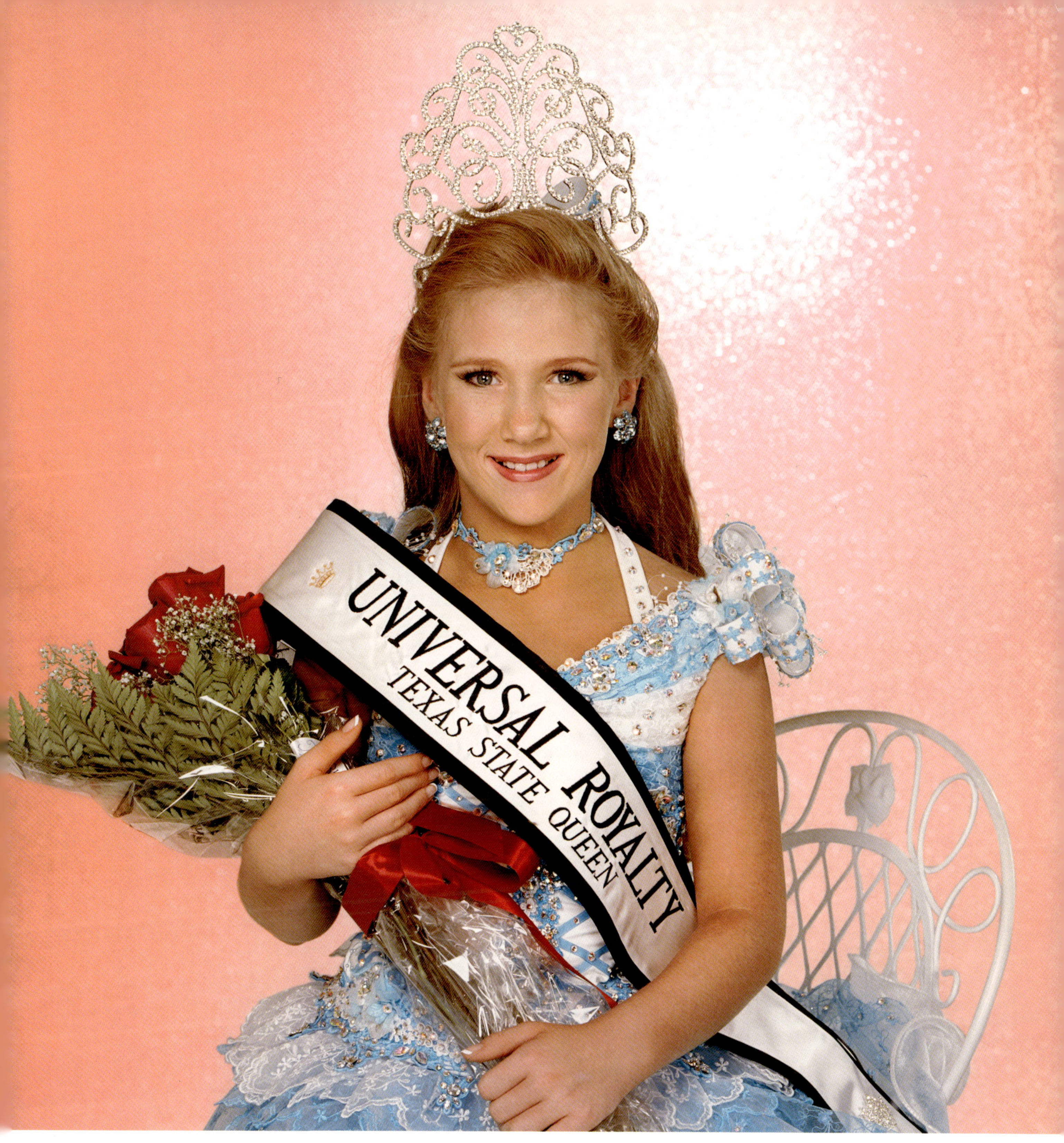

Elizabeth × Age 9 × Austin, Texas × 2005

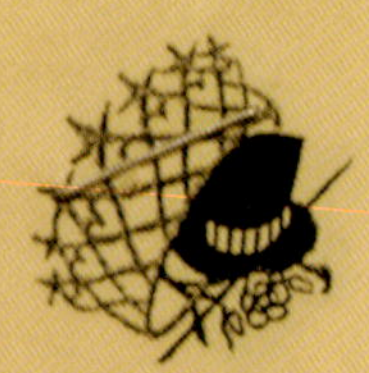

Official Score Sheet

Name: Lindsay # 50

Age: 6

Model

1.0 – 30.0	Facial Beauty	10
1.0 – 10.0	Poise	10
1.0 – 10.0	Personality	10
1.0 – 10.0	Over-all Package	10
	TOTAL	40

Comments:

______________ Judge

High Glitz Style Guide

with help from Kevin Posey

Beauty/Formal Wear

Talent

Pro-Am/Western Wear

Modeling

Hairstyles

Interview

Photogenic & Portfolio

Crowning

Titles

Beauty/Formal Wear

Beauty/Formal Wear is the signature event in a High Glitz pageant. Every little girl gets to dress up like Cinderella for the day. Contestants dress in custom, couture pageant gowns, with beyond extravagant hairstyles and high-octane makeup. A routine is done onstage, oftentimes in a T formation, that showcases the girl's outfit, hair, and beauty, as well as her poise and eye contact with the judges.

Elements of a Formal Wear outfit

Cupcake Ruffle Skirt: This skirt is made of varying types of fabrics, ranging from organza to raw-silk taffeta, and can utilize upwards of seven layers of fabric to create the shape of a cupcake piled to the top with decadent frosting, thus the name. When a skirt has all seven layers it's called a *full southern* evoking the gowns of debutante balls of yesteryear.

Older girls who compete in Glitz pageants wear longer Cinderella-style dresses.

Bodice: The bodice of a Formal Wear costume is usually constructed from Super Stretch nylon material, and can have boning and lacing much like a corset, in order to create an hourglass shape. This shell is then decorated with gemstones and other embellishments including satin or silk flowers, ribbons, lace and woven trim, marabou feathers, and bead work. These embellishments are sewn primarily by hand and this hand-sewn genius is known as *couture*.

Bustle: A bustle is a decorative "poof" of fabric that attaches to the bodice at the small of the back, resting delicately above the cupcake ruffle skirt, creating further dimension in form and shape. It is customarily designed with massive swags of fabric draped in various shapes such as bows or flowers.

Footwear: The classic High Glitz footwear consists of Mary Jane shoes, in white satin or patent leather. The shape of a traditional Mary Jane elongates the stride of anyone wearing them and being statuesque is never a bad thing in pageants. White anklets decorated with lace, ribbons, and/or bows complete and compliment the overall look.

Stance

Pretty Feet: Also called *model stance* or *Model T*, this stance mimics first position in ballet. The heel of the foot in front touches the inside arch of the other foot forming a "T." The hands are held out with straight elbows, and if the dress fits right, the fingertips just reach the edge of the cupcake skirt.

Talent

For the talent portion of the competition, contestants develop their own routines or work with a coach to develop an act that highlights their unique abilities. The costume worn should reflect the theme of the routine. Say the contestant chose a routine inspired by the old South. She could choose Dixieland music, an over-the-top costume, *Gone With The Wind*-style hair and makeup, and work the crowd like Scarlet trying to save the plantation.

As one seasoned pageant girl explained:

"Right now I'm doing tap dancing to a hip-hop and tap song. I've tapped and I've sung many different songs. Sometimes I do a commercial. I've done jazz dances, and all sorts of things. My favorite time though, was when I did monologue. I can't remember which pageant, but I winged it."

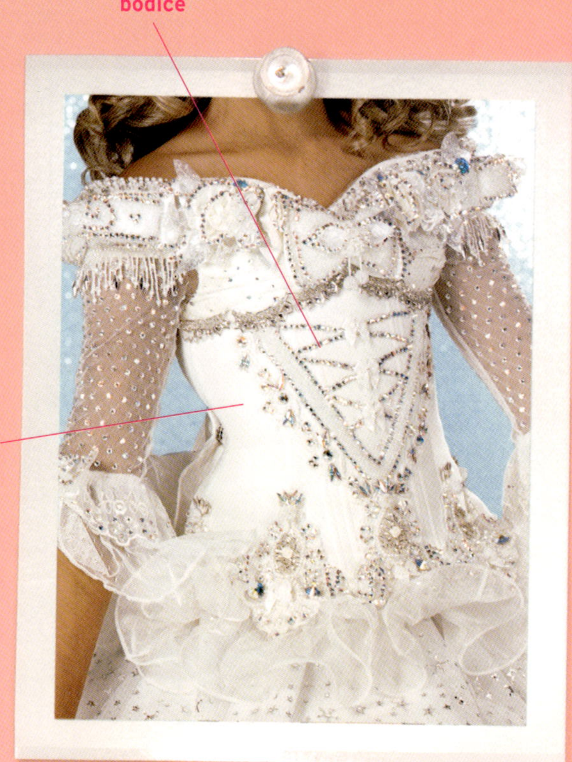

bodice

Super Stretch

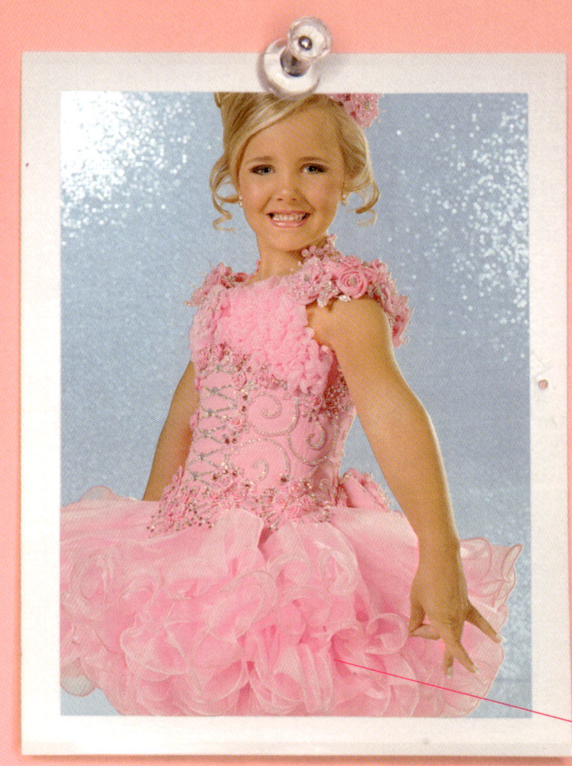

cupcake ruffle skirt

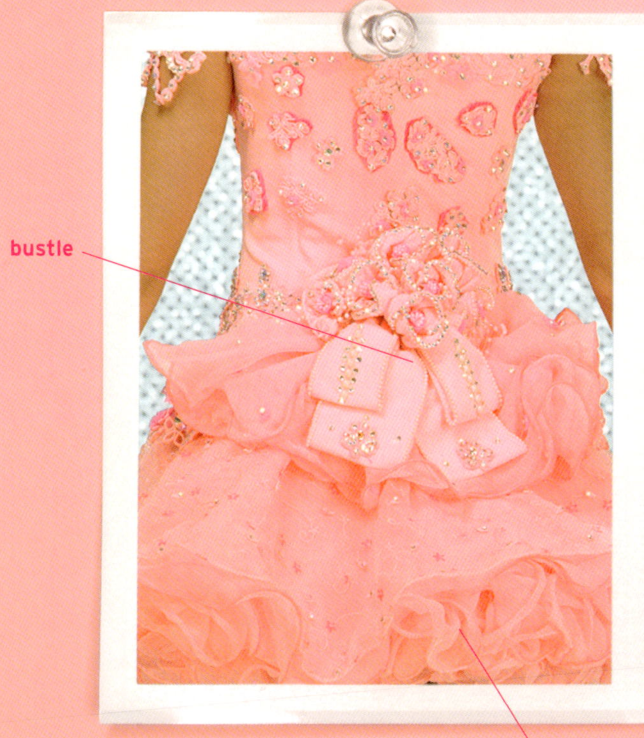

bustle

full southern

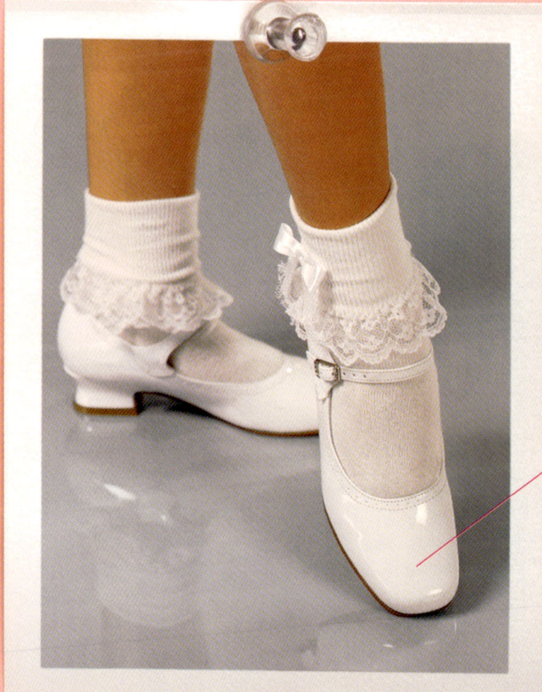

Mary Janes

pretty feet

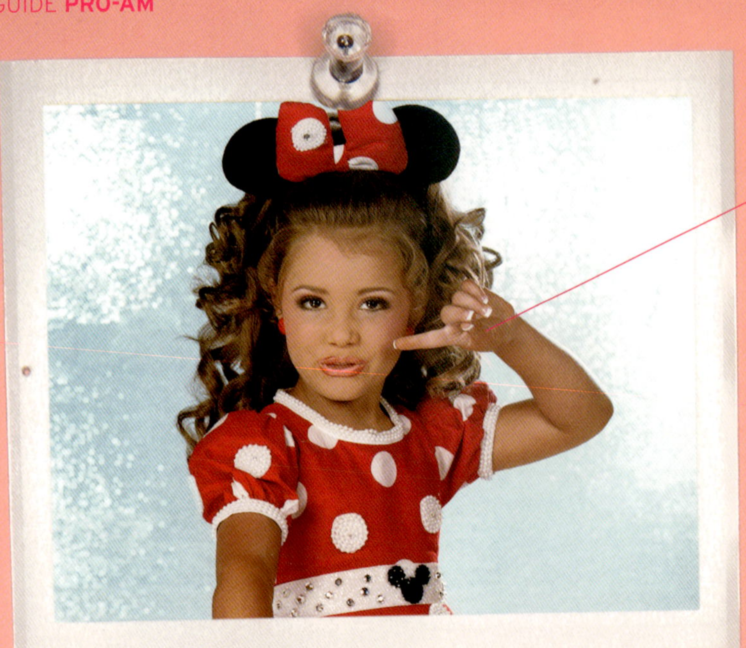

oohs and aahs

Theme Wear

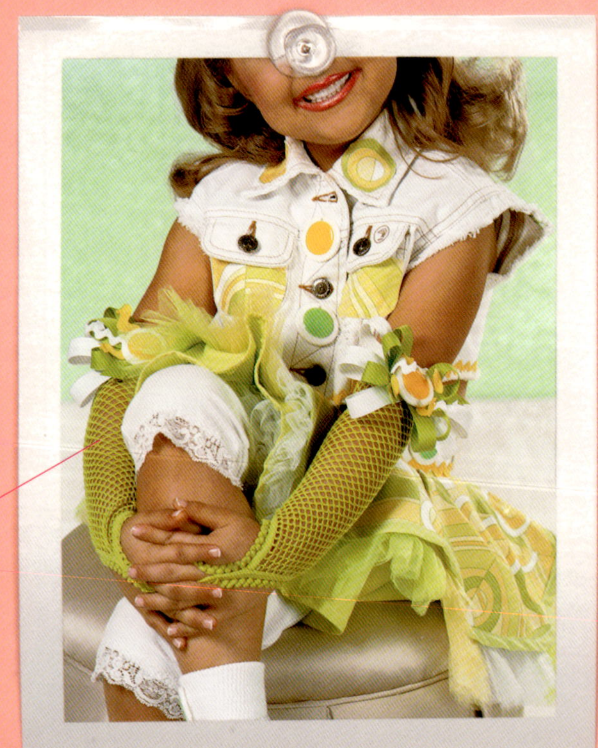

mesh

Sportswear

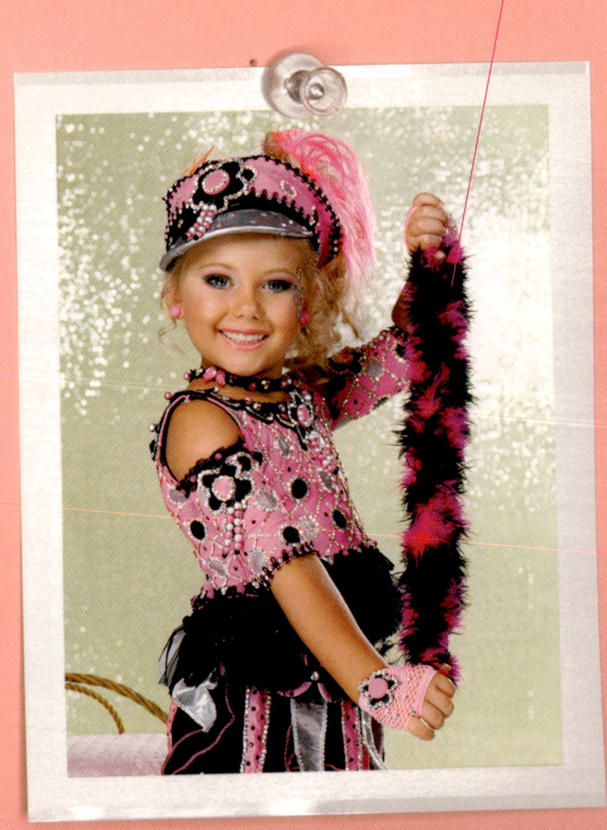

rip off

Pro-Am/Western Wear

Pro-Am outfits (a.k.a. Sportswear) are the most inventive and outrageous in pageantry. This is the full-on peacock moment! Costumes are covered in layers of ruffles, fringe, mesh, fur, feathers, beading, sequins, stones, and other decorations of all kinds. Bright-colored, metallic, and wildly patterned fabrics are used. These garments are often more body conscious and designed with embellished elements that move organically with the form. Pro-Am routines are a combination of dancing, vogueing (a quick series of poses performed as though modeling for a fashion magazine such as *Vogue*), and cheerleading. High-energy, club-mix, dance music is used as accompaniment. Some girls make up their own routines; others are developed with the assistance of a professional pageant coach.

Western Wear is the absolute tip-top in High Glitz glamour! From the meticulous detail of "liquid" beading to the strategic placement of fringe, it is hard not to recall the brilliant costumes created for Cher by the prolific fashion guru Bob Mackie. These costumes truly sparkle—just like those seen on the stage in Las Vegas.

Rip Off: This is a part of the garment that is usually attached to the shoulder or around the waist of the costume. It is then removed during the routine, and used as a prop to twirl around. The rip off can also be an entire layer of a costume. For example: when, at the end of a catwalk, a supermodel is showing off a full-length coat and removes it to reveal something even more amazing underneath. It can be made of fur or feathers, be a cape, skirt, shell, anything.

Oohs and Aahs: refers to facial expressions and gestures girls make during Pro-Am and Modeling routines. I like to think of these gestures as the punctuation at the end of a sentence!

Modeling

The modeling competition is similar to runway modeling. Done onstage with upbeat music, girls show off their garments and project, smile, and make eye contact with the judges. It's much like the glamour-soaked runways of Milan or Paris where the world's biggest supermodels strut their proverbial stuff in front of the glitterati elite. There are several different types of outfits suitable for Modeling, including Theme Wear such as *retro styles* and *red, white & blue*.

The wardrobe for Modeling is very different from the Beauty, Pro-Am, or Talent portions of the competition. Stylish and tasteful casual wear (or as they say in the fashion world ready-to-wear) off-the-rack and custom-made outfits are the ticket. A garment worn for Modeling could be donned on the street without drawing too much attention. No stones, sequins, glitter, or bling of any kind is allowed.

1950s retro styles are popular, characterized by graphic patterns such as polka dots, and full skirts with crinoline, to give that extra special kick to the swing of the garment. Imagine poodle skirts here!

"Red, White & Blue" can also be a category for modeling wardrobe in some pageants. Patriotic music is often used to accompany the R,W&B modeling category. Betsy Ross created the first American flag with embellishments in the shape of stars! It's nice to have the contestants pay homage to Old Glory in a way that would make Betsy proud.

Sometimes a Swimwear routine is similar to Modeling, but depending on the pageant, Swimwear can include more choreographed routines. Tasteful and age-appropriate swimsuits enhanced with rhinestones, flowers, ribbons, bows, ruffles, and other embellishments are worn.

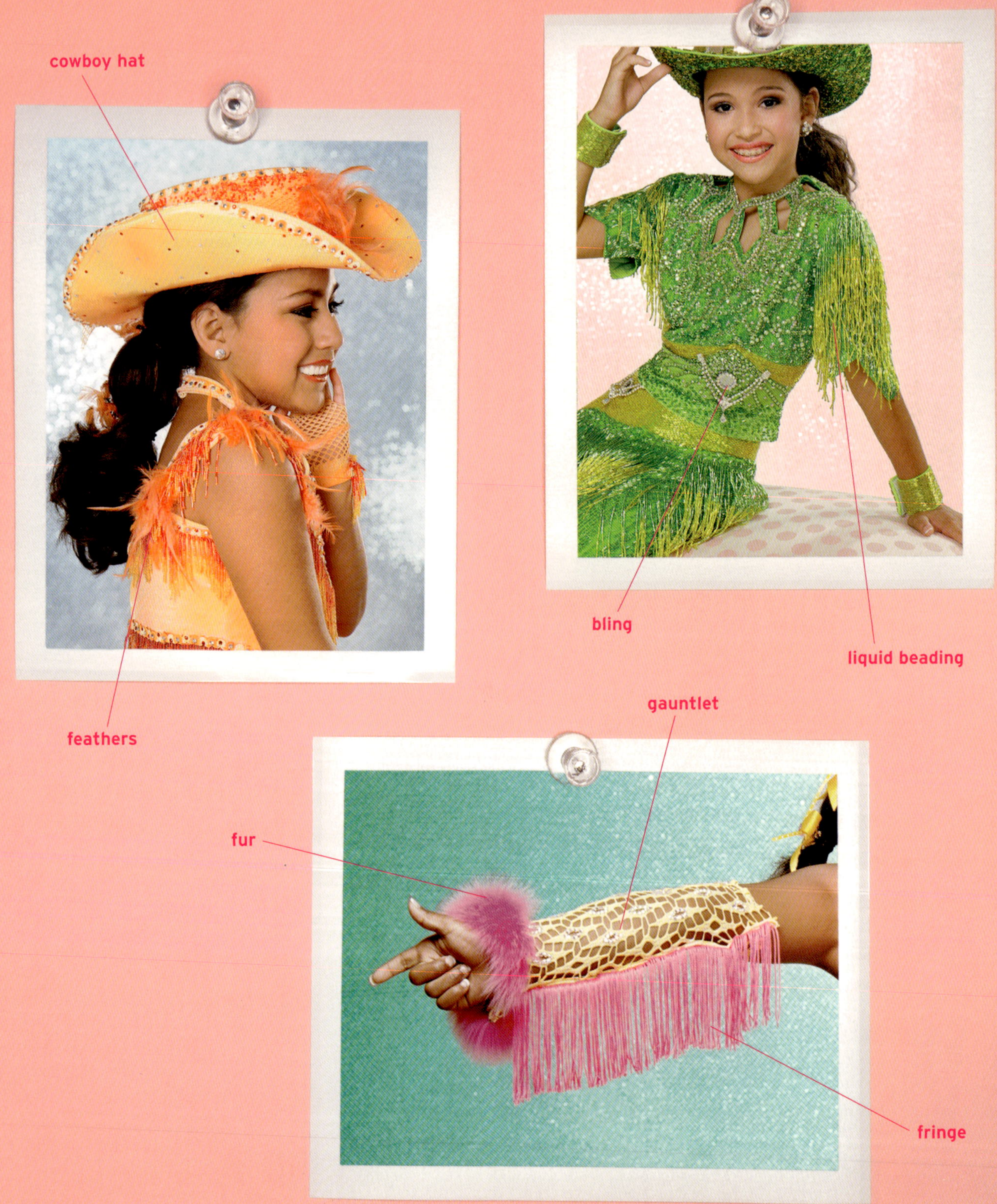
cowboy hat
bling
liquid beading
feathers
gauntlet
fur
fringe

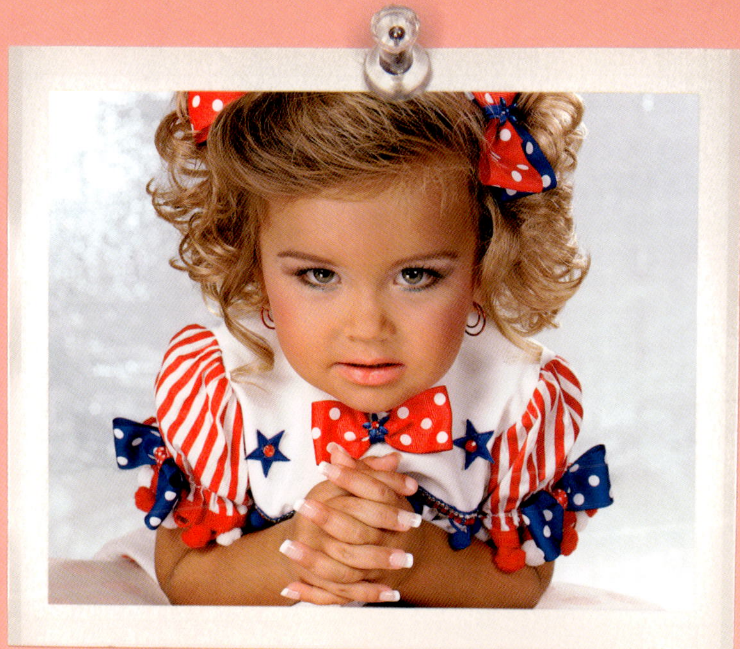

red, white & blue

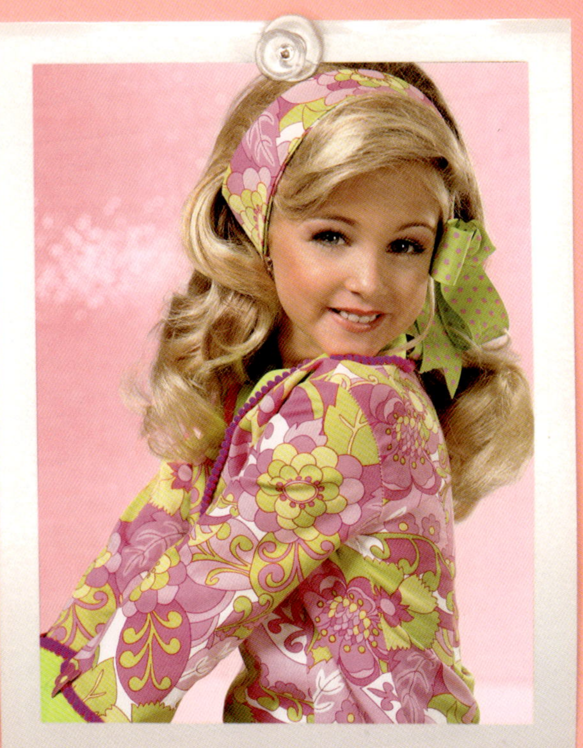

no bling

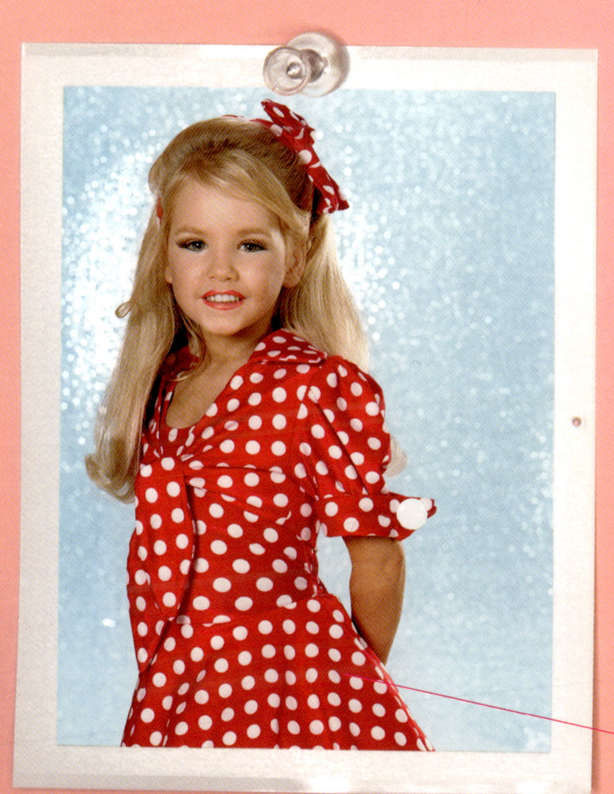

1950s

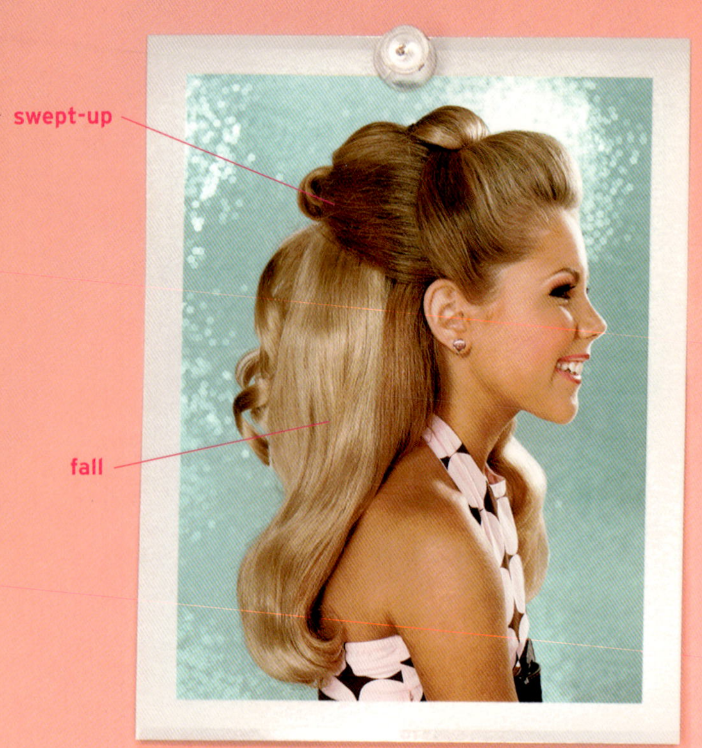
swept-up
fall

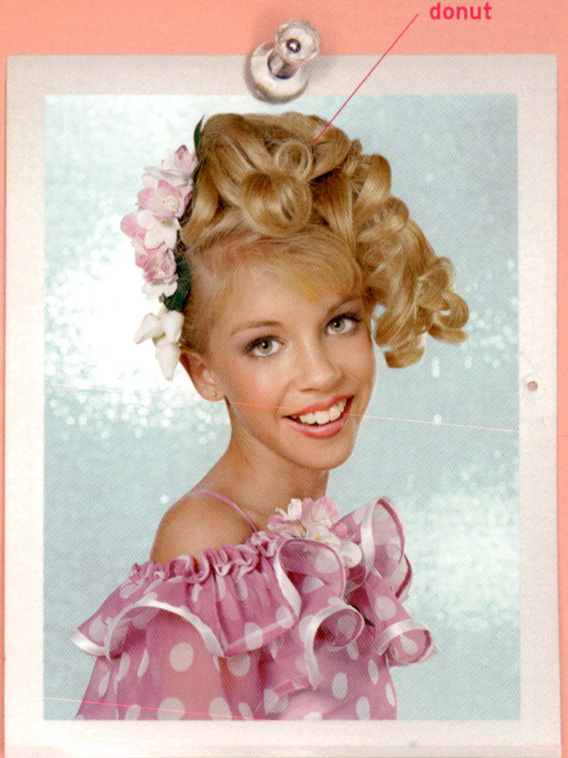
donut

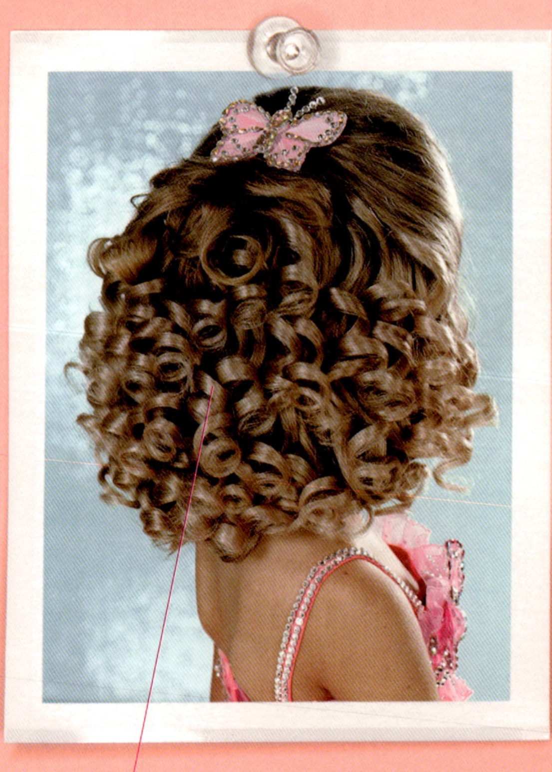
ringlets

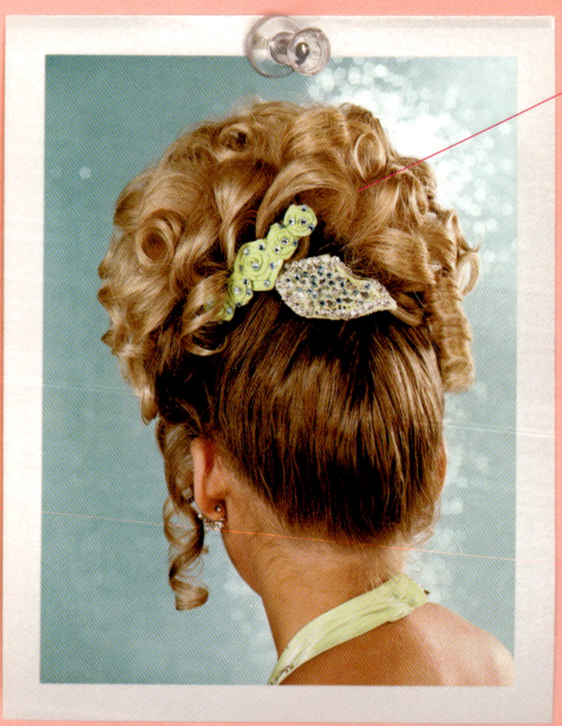
wiglet
up-do

Hairstyles

High Glitz hairstyles are sculptural works of art. Drawing their inspiration from as far back as Victorian ringlet curls to as current an up-do as one might see on the red carpet at the Oscars.

Oftentimes, professionals who specialize in pageant styles are hired to construct the competition creations. There are several key types of hairstyles, and variations on them.

Barbie: Blown out and tucked under or flipped under in back. This is a very mod, yet classic style in an understated, Jackie O kind of way (see page 143).

Up-do: Up-do's can be as simple as a French twist or as ornate as multi-layered chignon on the nape of the neck. The use of a hair donut adds height to a do when combined with add-ons. This is where individuality truly shines through.

Ringlets: Hairstyles featuring cascades of ringlet curls. Adding a ringlet extension or wig to the contestant's existing hair not only adds dimension, but also adds a stylistic twist that can compliment the shape of the outfit.

Swept Up: Combination of long hair and a towering crown. The modern-day beehive with a little something special flowing down the back. Inspired by styles of the 60s. Think Goldie Hawn on the go-go cube circa *Rowan & Martin's Laugh-In*.

Add Ons: Hairpieces such as wiglets, wigs, falls, and braids are added to create depth, define texture, give height, and generally enhance the shape of the face—sometimes framing it like a work of art.

Accessories: In Glitz pageants, one can never have too many accessories. So why not add them to the hairstyle for that extra bit of visual interest?

Interview

Frequently the interview takes place the night before the pageant competition. Participants are required to meet with three or four pageant judges to answer questions based on their bio. These are conducted either onstage or in a private room at the hotel where the pageant is taking place. No costumes or makeup are worn for this part of the competition.

The bio can include the contestant's name and age in addition to listing items such as: favorite hobbies, favorite foods, favorite TV shows, talents, and hopes and dreams.

"They might ask you an off-the-wall question," one veteran pageant contestant said. For example, "If you were to do something with Donald Trump's hair, what would you do? Would you dye it another color or flip it over to the other side?" or "When you are nervous onstage, what do you do to calm your nerves?"

Photogenic & Portfolio

Contestants are judged on a headshot or comp card (a printed card that shows various looks of the subject) that is submitted for the Most Photogenic competition. Judges review all submissions and award winners in each age group. Glitz photographs are digitized or enhanced by professional retouchers, who create the very polished and stylized type of portrait that often wins.

All of the big pageants have a category in the competition for photo portfolios.

The portfolio can include glitz portraits, natural portraits, composite images with fantasy themes, modeling comp cards, studio shots, and location photographs. To win, it helps to have an imaginative presentation and a good variety of photographs. Just like in the glamorous world of high fashion, when a model must visit a designer for a "go-see" to show their "books," this demonstrates versatility and the contestant's ability to convey many different styles.

Crowning

The crowning ceremony takes place after the competition, once the judges have tabulated the scores. The big winners in the pageant will be crowned onstage, before the entire audience, and oftentimes win cash, bonds, or cars in addition to their title, tiara, and embroidered satin sash. For the following year, until the next pageant takes place for the same pageant system, they are considered Reigning Royalty.

The Overall Package or the Total Package: This means you have all the right stuff to win the biggest title in the pageant. As one pageant flyer announced for the beauty competition:

"We are looking for a total package contestant. A beautiful face, clothes that fit well, and a wonderful personality. You will be judged on facial beauty, attire, personality, and stage presence."

Titles

Titles vary between circuits. The following titles, or variations of them, will be given out in most pageants.

Grand Supreme: The Grand Supreme is the ultimate title in any beauty pageant. It is awarded to the one contestant with the highest combined score in the pageant. The categories required to win this title vary from pageant to pageant. This is the shining star they are all shooting for—the title that carries the big prizes.

There can also be a Supreme title for the individual categories in the pageant. For example: Talent Supreme, Swimwear Supreme, Pro-Am Supreme, and Glitz Photo Supreme.

Mini Grand Supreme: This title is awarded to the next girl in line for the Grand Supreme title. She is the first runner-up for the biggest title in the pageant.

Divisional Supreme: This is the contestant with the highest combined score in her age group in the pageant.

Beauty Queen: One girl in each age group in a pageant will win the Beauty title for her division. The judges then select just one of these Beauty winners to determine the Overall Most Beautiful girl in the pageant, which is a more sought after title. The Most Beautiful girl is selected based on overall highest beauty score, but can also be the judges' preference.

Queen of Queens or Royalty of the Year: Some pageants will award one of these titles to the girl who earns the most points while representing her title and the pageant system that awarded it at various public events. This can include community service, hosting a parade, appearing at a preliminary or regional pageant, being introduced in her crown and banner at a public event, etc.

Lifetime Queen of Queens: This is an honorary title awarded to a retiring pageant girl, or to a girl who has competed in a pageant system and won many titles over the years. It can also be given to a girl whose family has worked hard for a pageant system over many years. This contestant will then be a permanent member of that pageant system's Royal Court.

Flippers: false front teeth veneers.

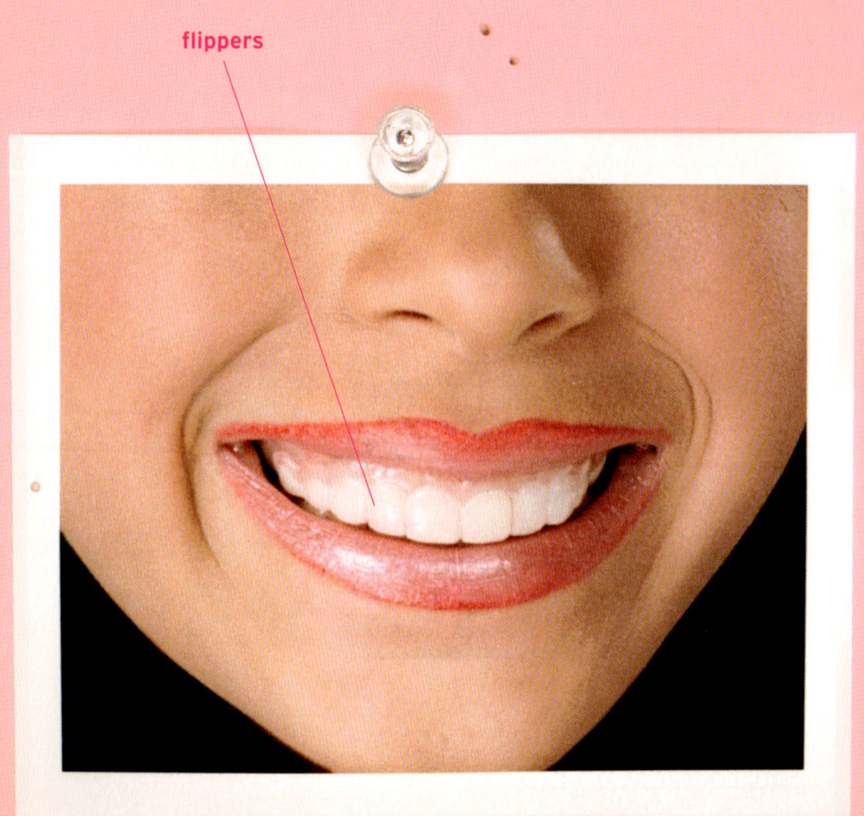
flippers

Thanks & Acknowledgements

The author would like to thank all of the girls and their parents who participated in this project, those published herein, and those not. I wish you all the best in pageants and in life. I am grateful to The Universal Royalty, Miss Royal Essence, Universal Miss & Masters International, and Dixieland Dolls & Darlings Beauty Pageants, and their directors. A heartfelt thanks to my literary agent, Stephen Frasier at Jennifer de Chiara Literary Agency NYC, who has been enthusiastic about this project from the start. To Craig Cohen, my editor at powerHouse for having the vision to select this book out of many to publish. Daniel Power, Will Luckman, and Sara Rosen also at powerHouse. Big thanks to my lawyers Alan Harris & Marcella Ruble, your support is invaluable. To Kopeikin Gallery in Los Angeles for being the first to represent this work, and for having the nerve to do it, I can't thank you enough. Deep gratitude to Adriaan van der Have, and TORCH gallery in Amsterdam, for giving me my first solo exhibition. The TORCH-Meister lives! And to Mo van der Have, for his continued success with TORCH. Thank you to the collectors who have purchased my works, and have made completing this project a reality. I am indebted to Liska + Associates, and Steve Liska, for taking on this project at a moment's notice, and for designing an absolutely stunning package for this book. To Liz Johnson for her creativity and attention to every detail of the design, and for keeping her sense of humor. Thank you Simon Doonan for accepting my invitation to write the foreword, I still laugh out loud every time I read it. My gratitude to Robert Greene who helped write my first book proposal, and contributed a thought-provoking introduction. Thanks to Tina and Lindsey George-Reyes for your pageant memorabilia and expertise. Kristin and Tina Cortines for the tiaras. Lisa Taylor for sharing her in-depth knowledge of pageants. Len Peltier for designing the book proposal that set the wheels in motion, Kevin Posey, Greg Collins, Sandra Kobrin and John Haskell for their creative input, Paul Elledge and Rocky Schenck. Thank you Autumn Lucas, aka Girl Friday, who was the ideal assistant. Leann Murphy for taking on Glitz in Nashville. Thanks go to my friends and family for their continuing encouragement, you know who you are! To everyone at A&I photo lab in L.A. and especially Baret Lepejian. Thank you Carole Thompson for championing this work early on, and Andy Schwartz for his help, and to Lucas the terrier for his patience and flawless artistry. Thanks Deborah Ayerst Artist's Agent and to Starpoint Studio in San Francisco, Vladimir Simovich, Michael Rochetti, and Matthew Triska. Finally, I want to express a special thanks to my parents Paul and Dorothy Anderson, who have always supported my creative endeavors. My father gave me my first camera when I graduated from High School, and I dedicate this book to his memory.

Katy × Age 5 × Las Vegas, Nevada × 2006

Lexi × Age 9 × Nashville, Tennessee × 2008 × (last page)

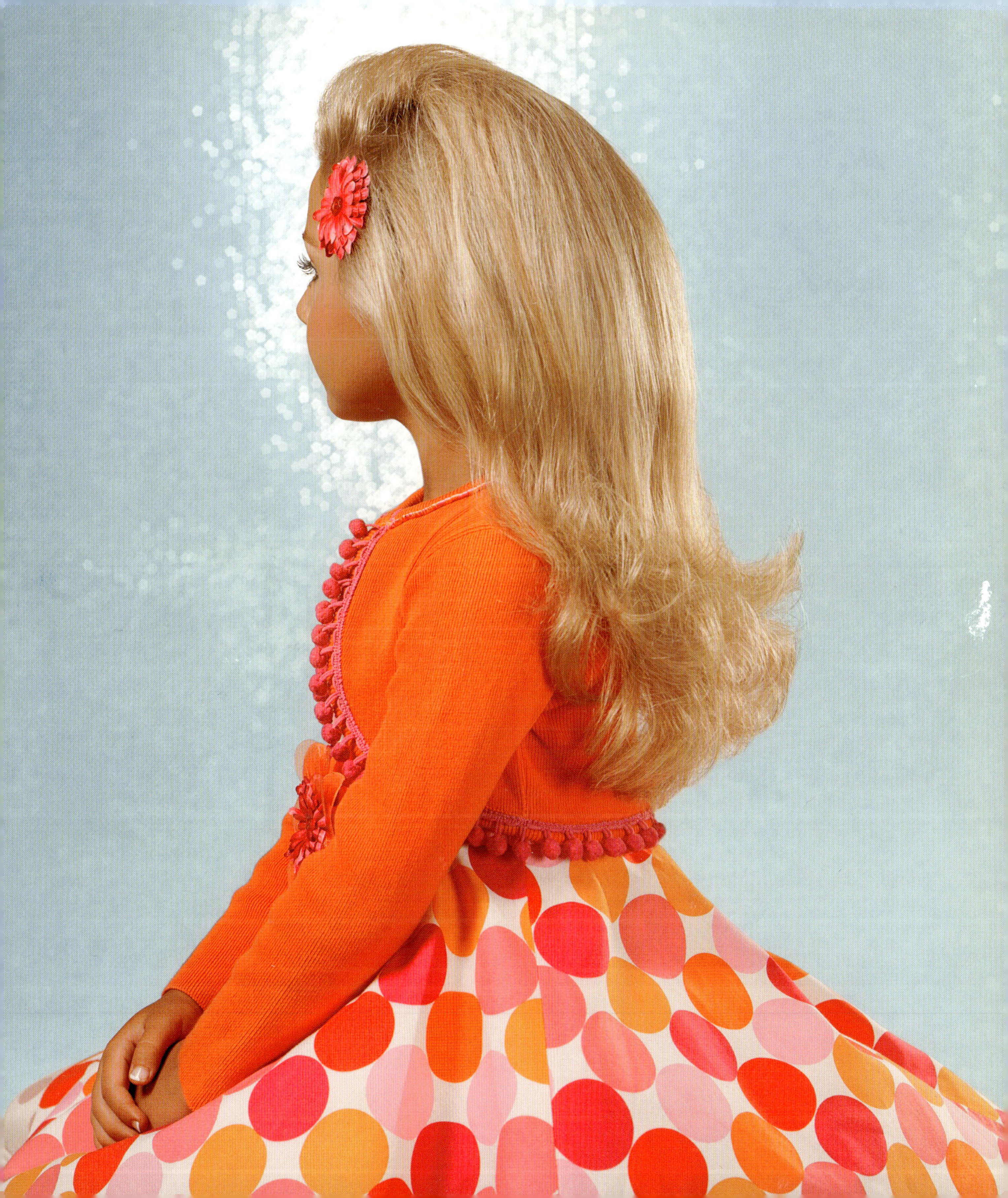

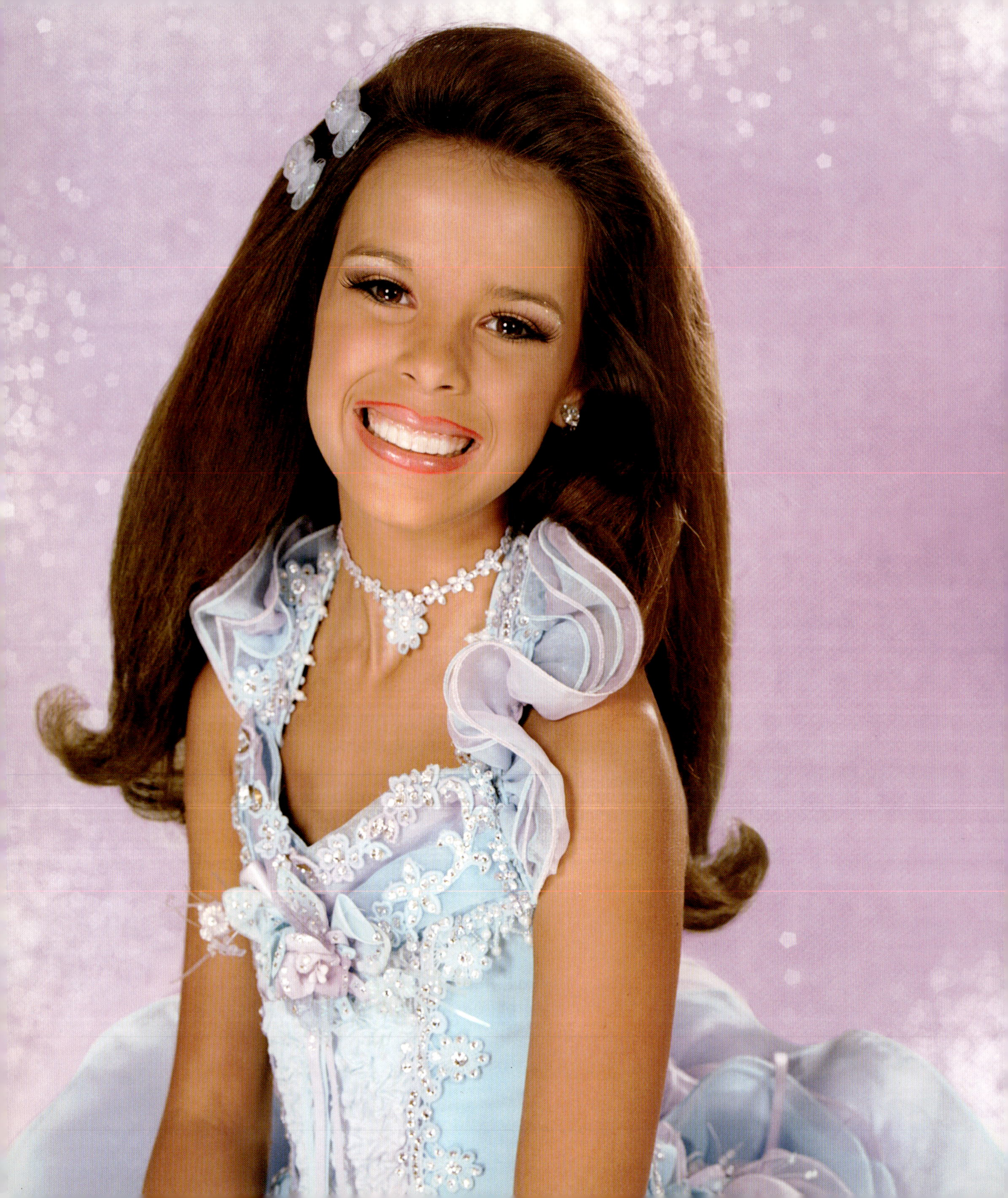

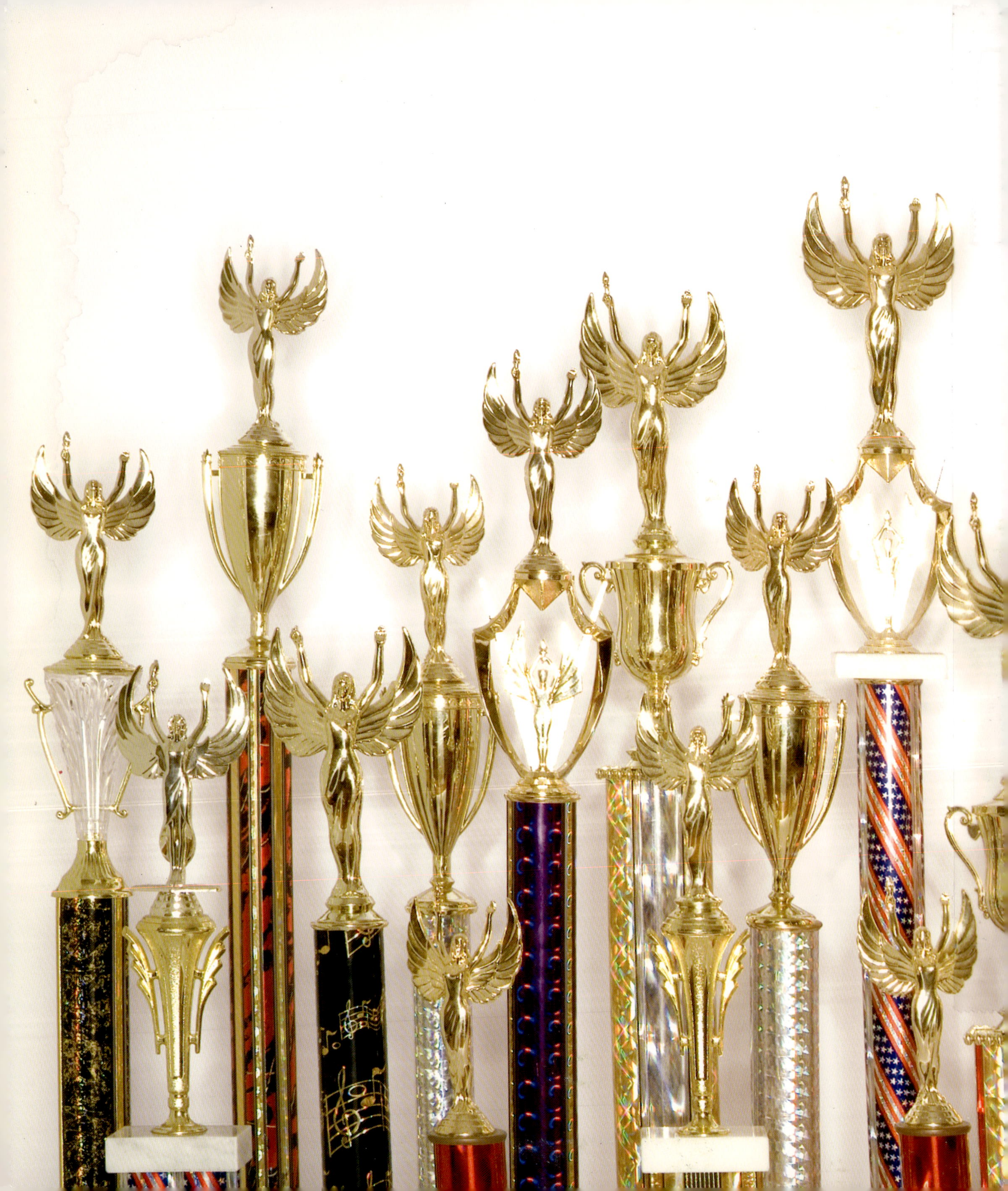